D1196229

PSYCHOLOGICAL VULNERABILITY

VULNERABILITY

C

TO

HRONIC
PAIN

Roy C. Grzesiak, PhD, is Assistant Professor and Co-Director of the Pain Management Center, Department of Anesthesiology, and Clinical Assistant Professor, Department of Psychiatry at the University of Medicine and Dentistry, New Jersey Medical School, Newark, New Jersey. He also serves as a Consultant to the Center for TMJ and Orofacial Pain Management at New Jersey Dental School on the same campus.

Donald S. Ciccone, PhD, is Assistant Professor of Psychiatry and Clinical Assistant Professor of Anesthesiology at the Pain Management Center, University of Medicine and Dentistry, New Jersey Medical School, Newark, New Jersey.

PSYCHOLOGICAL VULNERABILITY

TO CHRONIC PAIN

Roy C. Grzesiak, PhD
Donald S. Ciccone, PhD

Editors

Springer Publishing Company

Cover and interior design by Holly Block

Springer Publishing Company, Inc.
536 Broadway
New York, NY 10012

94 95 96 97 98 / 5 4 3 2 1

Library of Congress Cataloging-in-Publication Data

Psychological vulnerability to chronic pain / Roy C.
 Grzesiak, Donald S. Ciccone, Editors.
     p. cm.
   Includes bibliographical references and index.
   ISBN 0–8261–8070–1
   1. Chronic pain—Psychological aspects.   I. Grzesiak, Roy C.
 II. Ciccone, Donald S.
   [DNLM: 1. Pain, Intractable—psychology. WL 704 P9735 1994]
 RB127.P837 1994
 616'.0472'019—dc20
 DNLM/DLC
 for Library of Congress   94-6565
                                                                  CIP

Printed in the United States of America

To our children
Dina, Jim, and Dave (R.C.G.)
Leslie (D.S.C.)

Contents

Contributors

David J. Anderson, MD, is with Psychiatric Associates of San Francisco, San Francisco, CA.

Donald Bakal, PhD, is a Professor in the Department of Psychology at the University of Calgary, Calgary, Alta., Canada.

Stefan Demjen, PhD, is with the Division of Psychology, Foothills Hospital, Calgary, Alta., Canada.

Paul N. Duckro, PhD, is with the Division of Behavioral Medicine and the Department of Psychiatry and Human Behavior at Saint Louis University Medical Center, Saint Louis, MO.

Samuel F. Dworkin, DDS, PhD, is with the Department of Psychiatry and Behavioral Sciences, School of Medicine, and the Department of Oral Medicine, School of Dentistry, University of Washington, Seattle.

Yori (Yoram) Gidron is currently a PhD Candidate in Experimental Psychology in Behavioral Medicine at Dalhousie University, Halifax, N. S., Canada. He is sponsored, in part, by a Killam Scholarship.

Julie E. Goodman is currently a PhD Candidate in Clinical Psychology at Dalhousie University, Halifax, N. S., Canada. She is sponsored, in part, by a Studentship awarded by the Medical Research Council of Canada.

Robert H. Hines, MD, is with Psychiatric Associates of San Francisco, San Francisco, CA.

William G. Kee, PhD, is an Assistant Professor in the Department of Physical Medicine and Rehabilitation, Medical University of South Carolina, Charleston.

Veronica Lenzi, MA, is a doctoral student in Health Psychology at Yeshiva University, New York.

Donna L. Massoth, DDS, MSD, PhD, is with the Department of Oral Medicine, School of Dentistry, University of Washington, Seattle.

Patrick J. McGrath, PhD, is Professor of Psychology, Pediatrics, Psychiatry, and Occupational Therapy at Dalhousie University, Halifax, N. S., Canada, where he also directs the Clinical Psychology PhD Program.

Susan J. Middaugh, PhD, PT, is Professor, Department of Physical Medicine and Rehabilitation, Medical University of South Carolina, Charleston.

John A. Nicholson, MD, is Assistant Professor, Department of Physical Medicine and Rehabilitation, Medical University of South Carolina, Charleston.

Leanne Wilson, PhD, is with the Department of Oral Medicine, School of Dentistry, University of Washington, Seattle.

Preface

This volume is the result of our combined experience in the treatment of patients with intractable pain. Interestingly, the two editors have arrived at similar conclusions about vulnerability on the basis of different theoretical frames of reference. We both work as clinicians on a pain management service and have observed that many of our patients bring to the clinical setting a wide variety of premorbid characteristics. In many cases, these characteristics have complicated their adjustment to injury or illness and directly or indirectly caused their disability.

There is little doubt that the pain associated with traumatic injury or acute illness can be either exacerbated or ameliorated by premorbid psychological factors. There are, for example, vast individual differences in pain tolerance for physically identical pain stimuli. It is also well known that patients who sustain comparable injuries often do not recover at the same rate. Human pain and injury are necessarily experienced within a psychological framework that gives both meaning or personal significance. In the Appendix of this volume, the reader will find the article by George L. Engel entitled " 'Psychogenic' Pain and the Pain-Prone Patient" reprinted in its entirety from a 1959 issue of the *American Journal of Medicine*. For practitioners and researchers with a psychodynamic bent, this article is considered a classic. We believe it is one of the earliest statements on psychosocial vulnerability to chronic pain, and within it lie the seeds for much of what is being reexamined today. Over the last decade, a number of prominent cognitive theorists have recognized the influence of unconscious processes on both adaptive as well as maladaptive behavior. Even such a staunch behaviorist as Fordyce has acknowledged the role of cognition in mediating the degree of patient "suffering." Emotional disturbance or suffering and self-defeating illness behavior are the primary symptoms of chronic dysfunctional pain. However, we do not mean to imply that an unconscious "need" to suffer motivates all patients with chronic pain, for that certainly is not the case. An array of nonorganic factors may complicate recovery following a painful injury or illness. Some of the more common factors include economic disincentives; job dissatisfaction; mental impairment; premorbid psychiatric illness (including alcoholism and substance abuse); premorbid hypochondriasis or somatization; and a history of childhood trauma or illness. All of the above are capable of complicating the patient's response to medical intervention and/or prolonging the course of his or her pain syndrome.

Obviously, not all individuals with persistent pain engage in excessive or inappropriate illness behavior. What psychological or psychosocial events cause unnecessary or prolonged disability in certain individuals? It was with this question in mind that we asked a number of prominent scientist-practitioners to address the question of risk and vulnerability. In Chapter 1, Grzesiak offers a primarily theoretical view of symptom formation based on what he calls the matrix of vulnerability. He posits that vulnerability to pain-proneness or suffering is largely an unconscious process that has its origins in early developmental and/or psychosocial trauma. Knowledge of this trauma is typically dissociated, and it is only in the aftermath of new trauma (be it illness, injury, or disease) that there is a growing awareness of earlier episodes of suffering. Grzesiak attempts to integrate Engel's concept of pain-proneness with Melzack's concept of the neuromatrix to explain how psychological factors can complicate and, in some cases, actually perpetuate physical sensation as a consequence of one's identity as a suffering person. By combining psychodynamic thinking, trauma theory, and neurobiology, Grzesiak attempts to extend some of Engel's early ideas about vulnerability (see Appendix).

In Chapter 2, Dworkin, Wilson, and Massoth tackle somatization as a risk factor for chronic pain. In the context of chronic pain, they note that Somatization Disorder (as defined in the DSM III-R) is a rarity. However, somatization as a process is quite often part of the clinical picture for patients with chronic pain. According to these authors, somatization comprises two domains: (1) a perceptual-cognitive predisposition and (2) a behavioral predisposition toward symptom reporting and health care utilization. Although a possible link between somatization and depression is noted, they also address the cognitive-behavioral hypothesis that chronic dysfunctional pain may be an expression of nonspecific psychological disturbance. Although not all patients with chronic pain are somatizers, when somatization does occur in combination with chronic pain, there is a greater incidence of disability and utilization of health care resources.

In Chapter 3, Middaugh, Kee, and Nicholson examine the roles of muscle overuse and posture as factors leading to the development and maintenance of chronic musculoskeletal pain. They note that the largest increase in work-related musculoskeletal pain is not from isolated episodes of trauma but rather from cumulative trauma, repetitive strain, and muscle overuse. Rehabilitative efforts have generally focused on work site characteristics, and these authors emphasize the need to address operator characteristics as well. Their work demonstrates the innovative use of surface electrode electromyography (EMG) in both the assessment and treatment of musculoskeletal pain.

In Chapter 4, Goodman, Gidron, and McGrath address the concept of pain-proneness in children. They use the World Health Organization (WHO) model of the impact of chronic disease. The WHO model identifies four "planes of experience" by which the impact of pain can be assessed. The four planes are underlying cause, impairment, disability, and handicap. They apply the model to recurrent abdominal pain, headache and migraine, and dysmenorrhea. Vulnerability to pain-proneness is poorly understood in children. The authors suggest how future research can more appropriately address problems related to vulnerability and risk for chronic pain.

The problem of daily headache is addressed in Chapter 5. Bakal, Demjen, and Duckro note the importance of somatic awareness in the day-to day lives of individuals suffering from daily headache. Of particular note in their presentation is their observation that, for patients with chronic daily headache, many of the biobehavioral strategies that are routinely applied in the self-management of headache (such as ignoring early premonitory signs of pain) may actually aggravate the head pain. This is often further complicated by cognitive factors (negative expectations and beliefs) that add to overall headache-related impairment. They suggest that vigilance to preheadache warnings (somatic awareness) may provide a "window of opportunity" for self-regulation of headache. Although headache may reflect an inherited disposition involving central nervous system processes, they conclude that headache is still inextricably linked to affect and cognition.

In Chapter 6, Anderson and Hines draw on their years of experience with spine pain as well as their recent investigations of the interrelationships between childhood trauma, chronic back pain, and failure to successfully recover from spine surgery. They provide a psychodynamic explanation for susceptibility to chronicity and abnormal illness behavior. Their recent research has strongly suggested a link between early abuse, abandonment, parental addiction, and the potential for a chronic adaptation in the presence of spine pain. They use a psychoanalytic theory of attachment to explain how early psychosocial and/or developmental events, often trauma, can shape premorbid adaptation and lead to an inconsolability in the face of illness and pain.

Finally, in Chapter 7, Ciccone and Lenzi provide a critical overview of certain psychosocial variables that are thought to increase the risk of chronic pain following the onset of acute injury or illness. In their review they examine evidence that nonorganic factors may be responsible for causing or mediating disability behavior in certain individuals with chronic pain. Perhaps for the first time, they address factors as seemingly diverse as job dissatisfaction and childhood trauma in the context of psychological vulnerability. In addition, they consider the possibility that premorbid psychiatric illness, premorbid activity level, maladaptive thinking, and exposure to unhealthy reward contingencies may singly or in combination add to the patient's risk of chronic pain. They find that firm evidence linking *specific* psychosocial events with nonorganic disability is lacking at this time. They emphasize the need for both prospective and controlled retrospective investigations of selected psychosocial variables.

Chronic pain should not be thought of as a distinct diagnostic entity. Patients with chronic dysfunctional pain exhibit a variety of physical, behavioral, cognitive, and emotional problems that vary greatly from one individual to the next. Recent studies seem to show that psychological or nonorganic variables predict the patient's clinical course more accurately than so-called objective findings (such as MRI results). In other words, nonorganic factors seem to be responsible for actually "causing" certain individuals to become chronically disabled. The goal of this volume is to provide an introduction to the concept of psychological vulnerability and to suggest the variety of psychosocial variables that may be involved. It is hoped that the exploratory and admittedly speculative nature of this effort will have heuristic value and perhaps contribute to further exploration of this important subject.

ROY C. GRZESIAK
DONALD S. CICCONE
Newark, New Jersey
September, 1993

Chapter One

The Matrix of Vulnerability

Roy C. Grzesiak

Introduction

Since all the pain problems discussed in the following chapters are determined by multiple factors, including psychological ones, it is important to place psychological factors in context. At the outset, it should be noted that not all persons with persistent pain become chronic pain syndrome patients. Despite persistent pain, many individuals continue to love, work, play, and so forth without succumbing to disability lifestyle. What makes the difference? Who succumbs? Who copes well? Are there identifiable biopsychosocial factors that lead to chronicity? I think so. In fact, this volume is an effort to hone in on the biopsychosocial precursors of chronicity.

The scope of this chapter will be as follows. First, some of the evidence, both empirical and clinical, supporting the need for a more psychologically focused view of etiology, perpetuation and augmentation of chronic pain complaints will be presented. The value of a multiaxial approach to understanding pain will be demonstrated using a biopsychosocial model of stress-related symptom formation. Next, I will try to demonstrate just how psychological factors can fuse with biological processes to drive pain sensations toward chronicity. This argument will be accomplished by combining psychological theory, notably psychodynamic thinking, with advances made in our knowledge of central pain via both basic and clinical research in neuroscience. Finally, the utility of such an integration for our clinical work will be demonstrated. By combining some of the earliest writing on pain from a psychoanalytic perspective with concepts being put forward in contemporary neuroscience, I will attempt to demonstrate how a predominantly centralist position on the nature of pain can make sense of both our successes and failures in pain management. Furthermore, I shall attempt to demonstrate how the unique meanings of pain for each individual can be imposed on neural processes, leading to central reverberating patterns that operate in the absence of continuing peripheral afferent input.

It is suggested that the essence of vulnerability to chronic pain lies in a matrix of conscious and unconscious processes that promote suffering. In many cases, the unconscious factors have lain dormant, encapsulating or foreclosing the effects of early childhood trauma, until life events, usually physical or psychic trauma or illness, provide an avenue or theater for the expression of these long-hidden conflicts in chronic suffering (Grzesiak, 1992).

Acute Pain, Chronic Pain, and Chronic Pain Syndrome

Since most readers already have a working knowledge of the definitions of acute and chronic pain, only a brief review of them will be offered. One of the reasons for doing so is to underscore the somewhat idiosyncratic meaning I ascribe to chronic pain syndrome.

Acute pain is nociceptively driven pain; it is pain for which there is a readily available biological explanation. It is associated with trauma, illness, or disease. To the extent that there is an emotion associated with acute pain it is usually anxiety. In this context, anxiety makes sense because anxiety is a response to real or imagined threat to one's psychological or physical integrity. Acute pain should be treated aggressively by the physician, and there is no contraindication to using narcotic analgesics for pain relief. Most important, acute pain points the physician in the direction of proper diagnosis and treatment.

Chronic pain has none of the utility of acute pain. Chronic pain continues long after tissue damage should have healed, is frequently associated with depression, should not be treated with narcotic analgesics, and frequently must be managed because it is not amenable to relief (Tait, 1983). Using the guidelines of the International Association for the Study of Pain (IASP), it is suggested that pain that continues for more than three months should be considered chronic (Merskey, 1986). However, there are other views of chronic pain as well. Crue restricts the use of the term "chronic" to those pains for which no organic generator can be found (1978). If one restricts oneself to temporal guidelines, one risks a failure to appreciate underlying biological processes. Conversely, focus on biological processes often leads to a minimization of the concomitant or comorbid psychological domain. Failure to appreciate the importance of psychological factors in the person with acute pain can actually enable the movement toward chronicity.

Chronic pain syndrome is used in this context to refer to the person with persistent pain, regardless of etiology, who does not cope well and who succumbs to a broad array of biopsychosocial dysfunctions. Individuals with chronic pain syndrome do not function. They may no longer work, often rely excessively on pain medications or other psychoactive substances, subsist on workers compensation or disability income, make demands on health care services, and, for all practical purposes, are no longer leading meaningful lives. Unfortunately, these are the patients most often studied in pain clinics and, as Turk and Rudy (1990, 1991) have recently pointed out, are not representative of chronic pain patients as a whole. I would say that these samples primarily reflect individuals with chronic pain syndrome as opposed to the much larger sample of individuals who experience persistent pain. In two recent multiaxial studies it has been demonstrated that the psychological, as opposed to the biological, factors are most predictive of a chronic adaptation (Turk & Rudy, 1988; Rudy, Turk, Zaki, et al., 1989). A recent prospective investigation has strongly suggested that anxiety was the strongest predictor of chronic pain in a sample of herpes zoster patients (Dworkin, Hartstein, Rosner, et al., 1992). Thus, it is suggested that those who succumb to chronic pain syndrome bring to the clinical situation a vulnerability and a lack of resiliency somewhere within the biopsychosocial matrix. This kind of thinking has often led to volatile dialog in both the professional and pain patient community because it can easily be misconstrued as a "blame the victim" stance on chronicity. In fact, the idea that psychological factors may cause chronic pain syndrome is often interpreted as a "weakness" in the patient. Such an attitude reflects an inadequate understanding of the importance of mind-body interaction. As difficult as it may be to achieve for our diagnostic and therapeutic thinking, it is critical that we view symptom expression as the outcome of a multiply determined, and often synchronous, psychobiologic process. Chronic pain reflects the simultaneous expression of sensation and mood.

Pain and Suffering States of Mind

An alternative approach to defining pain has been suggested by Loeser (Loeser & Black, 1975; Loeser, 1982). Loeser has broken pain into its component parts; namely, nociception, pain, suffering, and pain behavior. *Nociception* refers to the potentially tissue damaging mechanical, thermal, or chemical energy impinging on a specialized nerve ending capable of initiating a pain signal transmission in the nervous system. *Pain* is the perception of that signal in the central nervous system. *Suffering* refers to the many unique, historical, and current idiosyncratic meanings the individual ascribes to pain and suffering. *Pain behavior* refers to the overt signs that tell the observer that this individual is in pain. I present this model here because, although Loeser meant it to define the parameters of the behavioral model, I wish to emphasize the importance of suffering in the overall clinical picture. Loeser (1982) also emphasized the fact that pain, suffering, and pain behavior can continue in the absence of nociception. This can be viewed from either a psychological or a neurological point of view. From a neurological perspective, the divorce of nociception from pain experience would indicate centralization of the pain. From a psychological perspective, it could reflect a conversion process as well.

One of the profound dangers in diagnostic work with chronic pain patients is the tendency to fall into a mind-body trap in which dualistic thinking mandates that we locate the origins of pain sensation either in the body or in the mind. For pains that have persisted for some length of time, that approach to diagnostic thinking is simplistic and often futile. This is not a new idea. Almost 100 years ago, in *Studies on hysteria*, when discussing the origins of Elisabeth von R's pain, Freud stated: "The circumstances indicate that this somatic pain was not *created* by the neurosis but merely used, increased and maintained by it. . . . There has always been a genuine, organically-founded pain present at the start. It is the commonest and most widespread human pains that seem to be most often chosen to play a part in hysteria" (Freud & Breuer, 1895). Similarly, in *Fragment of an analysis of a case of hysteria*, Freud made the observation that the motivation for maintaining a physical symptom may have nothing whatsoever to do with the mechanisms that caused the initial medical problem (1905). In this short vignette, Freud made an important point that remains germane for contemporary psychosomatic diagnosticians, namely, that intractable physical symptoms can be divorced from their original biological origins.

This is consistent with contemporary diagnostic thinking. For example, in the *Diagnostic and Statistical Manual of Mental Disorders* (DSM-III-R, 1987), the use of the diagnosis Somatoform Pain Disorder does not require an absence of physical findings but can be used when the physical complaints and related social or occupational impairments are far in excess of what one would expect given the nature of the physical findings. In clinical work with chronic pain patients, it is often suffering (an affect), not pain (a sensation) that is the primary problem.

A Biopsychosocial Approach to Symptom Formation

One of the major stumbling blocks in pain management involves just how psychological processes work in the so-called mysterious leap from the mind to the body. Yes, there is a fancy metatheory of how conversion processes work, but to view all chronic pains as a consequence of hysterical conversion or somatization would be simplistic and inappropriate. There is a significant literature that suggests one must take contemporary life events into consideration as well. Over the last few years, I have worked more with chronic temporomandibular disorder (TMD) and orofacial pain patients and, in an effort to explain how their symptoms develop, have relied on a biopsychosocial model of symptom formation that was initially developed by Wickramasekera (1986). This particular model was initially used to explain the interaction of biopsychosocial factors in stress-related symptom formation. However, I have found it useful as a way of trying to understand how patients come to be at a particular point in the course of their pain syndrome (Grzesiak, 1988, 1991a, 1991b). Furthermore, I find this model useful because it has an atheoretical flavor to it that allows for flexibility in clinical understanding and application.

Because Wickramasekera (1986) conceptualized his model as applying to *stress-related* disorders, including pain, it certainly cannot serve as a model for all pain-related symptoms. In a recent review of orofacial pain syndromes, I did find that one of the major life circumstances preceding or co existing with the onset or increase in pain symptoms was stress, the other was depression (Grzesiak, 1991b). In this context, I certainly believe Wickramasekera's model should be given thoughtful consideration within pain management.

In his model of symptom formation, Wickramasekera (1986) identified five categories of risk factors that he broke down into three subsets that were called predisposers, triggers, and buffers. As I present these risk factors, I will elaborate on the relevance for chronic pain syndromes.

Predisposers

The first three risk factors are viewed as predisposers; they are hypnotic susceptibility, catastrophic thinking, and sympathetic reactivity.

Risk Factor 1

High or low hypnotic susceptibility are both indicated as potential risk factors in symptom formation. Hypnotic capacity is a normally distributed individual difference trait with approximately 10% of the population falling at either extreme (Barber, 1969). It is important to note that this is not an endorsement for clinical hypnosis but rather an exposition of the fact that hypnotizability has a number of cognitive and perceptual dimensions that can contribute to symptom formation. Hypnotic susceptibility refers to a capacity to enter a dissociated state of mind. This dissociated state of mind may occur without formal hypnotic induction, as in the case of either severe trauma or extremely low psychological arousal. Experiences that are processed in a dissociated state of mind are subject to state dependency; in other words, they cannot be recollected unless the individual returns to that dissociated state of mind.

It is not uncommon to find symptoms of posttraumatic stress disorder (PTSD) in pain patients, particularly when the onset of a persisting pain is trauma-related. This explains the resistance of many PTSDs to psychological intervention and also makes it more understandable why hypnosis is often the treatment of choice for PTSD. For a clinical example of hypnosis in the treatment of pain in PTSD, see Dworkin and Grzesiak (1993, pp. 375–377).

Individuals who are high in hypnotic susceptibility are at risk for symptom formation for a number of reasons. These individuals have rich fantasy lives, a vivid capacity for imagery, the capacity to voluntarily hallucinate (not a psychotic process), an enhanced capacity for sensory memory, including pain and an exquisite sensitivity to mind-body nuance. They are more likely to experience physiological changes as a consequence of their thinking. They can produce imaginal changes in virtually all sensory systems. Placed in a situation of high or low stress, a situation that can activate a dissociated state, they are more likely to learn, remember and incubate the experience of acute pain. When placed under high or low stress again, they are more likely to reactivate previously experienced pains and fuse them with current difficulties. The importance of early trauma in memory functioning and in the compulsion to repeat trauma and to reenact and recreate traumatic or victimized roles has been well articulated by van der Kolk (van der Kolk, 1989; van der Kolk & van der Hart, 1991). Wickramasekera (1986) also makes the important observation that the activated state may involve either high or low arousal. Not surprisingly, these individuals are more prone to fears, phobias, and other anxieties.

Individuals who are low in hypnotic susceptibility are at risk for entirely different reasons. The quality of their thinking is very literal and concrete. They do not make connections between psychological events and physical responses. They tend to avoid, deny, or minimize somatic cues and, when placed in a traumatic situation, they tend to inhibit verbal, emotional, and behavioral response. This inhibitory problem-solving style brings with it an autonomic activation and increased risk for stress-related symptom formation (Pennebaker, 1985). Individuals who are low in hypnotic capacity often develop chronic symptoms because they avoid, deny, or misinterpret signals from their bodies. They also tend to avoid medical care and, therefore, frequently suffer unnecessary physical damage because of delaying appropriate medical care.

In recent years we have seen a resurgence of interest, along with some empirical studies, documenting the disproportionate number of chronic pain patients who have been victims of trauma, abuse, and loss during childhood (see, for example, Anderson & Hines, this volume). Since early trauma tends to be processed in an altered or dissociated state of mind and not brought into awareness until additional trauma occurs later in life, one could speculate about the interrelationships between early trauma, dissociative trends, hypnotic susceptibility, and psychosomatic vulnerability.

Risk Factor 2

Catastrophic thinking is the second risk factor for stress-related symptom formation. It, too, is a predisposing factor. Catastrophic thinking was initially defined by Ellis (1962) to explain certain psychopathological processes. Wickramasekera defines catastrophic thinking as "becoming intensely and frequently absorbed in a negative psychological or sensory event and talking to oneself about it in ways that potentiate its aversive properties" (1986). Catastrophic thinking contributes to pain exacerbation in a number of ways. Catastrophic thinking leads to increased anxiety (sympathetic nervous system activation) which, in turn, will lead to greater tension, preoccupation with symptoms, enhanced memories of pain and suffering, and so on. Ciccone and Grzesiak (1984) have also defined many of the cousins of catastrophic thinking; the important feature being the power of irrational beliefs to alter adaptation and, consequently, to increase the likelihood of pain-related disability. In addition to catastrophic thinking, the literature from behavioral medicine suggests that pessimism, self-doubt, passivity, and dependency are all modest predictors of stress-related and other psychosomatic disorders (Wickramasekera, 1986). Copers and catastrophizers appear to be at extreme ends of a continuum. In a study of somatization and pain complaint, Dworkin and associates speculated that: "Our data . . . are consistent with the possibility that both depression and somatization are linked to a common predispositional dimension of perceptual/cognitive style involving augmentation, catastrophizing and amplification" (S. Dworkin, Von Korff, & LeResche, 1990).

Risk Factor 3

Autonomic lability or neuroticism is a biological predisposer. Although it is somewhat difficult to understand the connection between autonomic lability and neuroticism, Eysenck viewed autonomic lability as one of the most significant physiological correlates of neuroticism (1983). Wickramasekera (1986) is referring to sympathetic reactivity and breaks this predisposer into two dimensions, namely, autonomic lability and autonomic response stereotypy. Autonomic lability refers to the degree of reactivity in subsystems of the autonomic nervous system. Both elevated baselines and delays in returning to baseline after stressing situations are correlated with physical complaints and stress-related disorders. Autonomic response stereotypy refers to the fact that individuals react to stress with characteristic and consistent patterns of response that may differ between individuals but not within individuals (Lacey, 1967; Sternbach, 1966). What this means is that individuals have a preferred autonomic system response or "weak link" that is activated when under stress. This explains the difference in symptoms between individuals undergoing relatively similar stress. Some react with headaches, some with back pain, some with palpitations, and so on.

Triggers

Risk Factor 4

Major life changes and multiple daily hassles constitute trigger factors for stress-related symptoms. The initial literature on major life changes was in the context of risk for cardiovascular illness (Holmes & Rahe, 1967). In recent years both major life changes and multiple daily hassles have been implicated not only for cardiovascular risk but for health problems in general. When one has a number of major life changes in a short period, there appears to be a higher probability of developing illness. Major life change would appear to be stressful in-and-of-itself because it involves attaining a new adaptation. However, it is important to remember that stress responses generally reflect coping failure. Coping involves the private appraisal of a situation as potentially threatening or harmful to one's well being (Lazarus & Folkman, 1984). Coping always requires reaching inside oneself for something extra, adaptation does not. While major life events have been implicated in health status for years, only recently have investigators documented the insidious effects of multiple minor daily hassles to health as well (Kanner, Coyne, Schaefer, et al., 1981; DeLongis, Coyne, Dakof, et al., 1982). Hassles typically involve psychosocial stressors that are more subtle, insidious, and intermittent but that are unrelenting. Some examples would be noise, work overload, aging parents, problem children, and so forth. Often these factors cannot be changed in any meaningful fashion, so clinicians must work at changing the impact of the person's appraisal of them so as to delimit the potential deleterious effects on health.

Buffers

Risk Factor 5

The final area of psychosocial risk involves *social support systems and coping skills*. Essentially, people serve as buffers to the stress response. There is an accumulating literature on the importance of other people to one's health and adaptation. It is important to know that you have someone you can talk to about the stresses of your day, be it a friend, spouse, or lover. Coping skills are an important determinant of what the effects of daily activities, life changes, painful illness, etcetera will be on our health. The coping skills dimension of this buffering factor interacts with Risk Factor 2, catastrophic thinking. Consequently, what one thinks about one's situation can help or hurt adaptation to stressful events, shape stress-related symptom formation, and determine outcome after the development of stress-related or painful illness.

The biopsychosocial model proposed above can enable clinicians and researchers who work with pain patients to have a better understanding of how a wide variety of events and processes can interact, leading to pain and disability or turning the person toward a reasonable adaptation. This model is particularly helpful in explaining the interaction of predisposers, triggers, and buffers in determining the ultimate symptom picture. However, although Wickramasekera (1986) calls them risk factors, which they may in fact be in the case of many of the stress-related disorders, in the presence of persisting pain, these factors may be more appropriately viewed as perpetuators. For example, catastrophic thinking is not likely to *cause* pain but such thinking certainly can serve as the generator through which a persisting pain turns into a chronic-pain syndrome.

When one is confronted with a patient who seems to embrace pain and suffering, the so-called pain-prone individual, a more comprehensive model is needed. It must be a model that can accommodate issues of personality, unconscious processes, and suffering. The model I am about to propose represents an attempt to integrate Engel's psychodynamic position with the advances made in neurobiology as it relates to pain (1959). This venture is not an attempt to create a new theoretical model; it is an attempt to take what is already known about the psychological aspects of pain, particularly factors that play to vulnerability for suffering states of mind, and integrate them with the newer findings stemming from neuroscience, most notably, the work of Melzack (1989, 1991, 1992) on the neural substrates of pain. From this integration, I believe we have a clinically useful explanation for how some individuals fail to recover from painful illness and trauma, succumb to pain-related suffering, develop disability lifestyles, and never come to a reasonable adaptation to their persisting pain.

The Signature Concept

The concept of signature to describe or mark the identity of a particular object was first used in psychiatry by George Engel. In 1959, Engel wrote what is in the minds of many psychodynamically oriented practitioners, a classic article on the nature of psychogenic pain and pain-proneness. This particular publication has been generally ignored by the last two generations of behaviorally and cognitive-behaviorally focused pain psychologists. Engel, an internist trained in psychoanalysis, was attempting to understand the nature of so many of his patients who had long-standing pain without clear-cut or identifiable pathophysiology to account for the problem. In his attempt to understand so-called psychogenic pain, Engel spoke of the *peripheral signature* and the *individual psychic signature*. To these two signatures, which will be defined below, I would like to add the *neural signature*. Drawing from the work of Melzack on the neuromatrix (1989, 1991, 1992) and Melzack and Loeser, (1978), I would suggest that the neural signature is a dynamic composite of current peripheral signatures and both the current and the historical psychic signature.

The Peripheral Signature

Engel (1959) defined the peripheral signature as referring to the relatively good concordance between the patient's description of the pain and what the physician knows about somatopathologic processes capable of producing pain. In other words, the description of the pain has diagnostic utility; by virtue of its pattern, location, intensity, and quality, the physician is led to an accurate diagnosis. Aberrant anatomical and physiological processes in any given system typically present a distinct and predictable kind, duration and intensity of pain. Classical examples of pains from the periphery are in medicine the lower-quadrant abdominal pain and rebound tenderness associated with an inflamed appendix and in dentistry, the all-consuming ache and exquisite temperature sensitivity found in caries. Engel explained that although such classical patterns are "common knowledge, I stress it because the precise elucidation of such correlations between anatomical and physiological characteristics on the one hand, and pain experience on the other hand, provides the most certain evidence that processes originating in the periphery are initiating a particular pain experience" (1959, p. 903). He went on to warn physicians that deviations from these known patterns should not be too quickly labeled atypical but that some consideration should be given to the possibility that the pain, originally a peripheral signature, has taken on additional meaning and purpose.

Accurate determination of the peripheral signature is the purview of the physician or dentist. The determination of anatomical and physiological concordance does not belong within the domain of psychological practice. In pain management, one of the only exceptions I would offer to this would involve musculoskeletal pain wherein the psychologist with training and expertise in psychophysiology conducts surface electromyographic muscle scanning to identify aberrant patterns of muscle activity and function (e.g., Middaugh & Kee, 1987; Ciccone & Grzesiak, 1990; Middaugh, Kee, & Nicholson, Chapter 3). Generally, determination of the biological or physical cause of any particular pain problem lies with the physician, dentist, or physical therapist members of the pain management team. Because psychologists have little to offer in identifying the peripheral signature, it will not be given further attention here.

The Individual Psychic Signature

Private meanings ascribed to pain, illness, and suffering contribute to the individual psychic signature. All aspects of the patient's description of pain that do not fit or concur with the peripheral signature can be assumed to fall within the individual psychic signature. Engel offered that "in general, the more complex the ideation and the imagery involved in the pain description, the more complex are the psychic processes involved in the final pain experience" (1959, p. 904). Yet Engel cautioned practitioners that it must not be assumed that the patient who gives us complex and confusing descriptions of pain does not have a peripheral lesion. The individual psychic signature has the capacity to obscure the peripheral signature and can lead to the erroneous conclusion that the pain problem is essentially psychogenic which, of course, then results in inappropriately psychologically oriented treatment.

Engel believed that the individual psychic signature could carry a pain proneness that has its origins in early developmental experiences. At this juncture, I would like to emphasize the fact that Engel did not imply that there existed a singular or unitary pain-prone personality; rather, he believed that there were pain-prone personality patterns found within a number of personality types and character organizations.

Just how can early developmental experience impact on psychological functioning to impart a propensity for pain proneness? Engel outlined six ways in which pain and developmental experience interact to provide idiosyncratic meaning to the individual psychic signature for pain and suffering.

1. Pain serves as a warning of imminent or real body damage or loss. As such, it is intimately connected to learning and environment; we learn the dangers of the environment and the limitations of our bodies. Equally important, according to Engel (1959), we can assume that these early pains are permanently registered in the body as "pain memories" and become part of a "body pain image." Since all pains are stored in memory, retrieval is possible and, clinically, we often find that earlier pains become mixed with current injuries complicating the patient's clinical presentation.
2. Developmentally, Engel (1959) pointed out that pain is inextricably tied to human relationships. Early in infancy, the baby learns that crying will bring a response from a loved one or caretaking person. Pain brings with it the anticipation of reunion with a love object. Depending on the kind of parenting or caretaking the baby receives, a pain focus will be more-or-less a part of its adult character. We must, of course, add to this early learning of the communicative value of pain the important work of Fordyce over the years (e.g., 1976) on the contingencies or rewards that can come to an individual because of displays of pain behavior.
3. Early in childhood a link is established between pain and punishment. In other words, as Engel stated, "pain is inflicted when one is bad" (1959, p. 901). Closely associated with the notion of badness is the experience of guilt. Tying these concepts together, pain can serve as expiation for guilt over real and/or imagined shortcomings.
4. Pain is associated with aggression and power. It does not take the child long to learn the untoward consequences of inflicting pain on others or on himself. Pain can serve to contain one's own aggression by channeling that aggression into oneself, or at oneself.
5. According to Engel (1959), a closely related concept is the association of pain and real, threatened, or fantasized loss of

loved ones. As we shall see in a later example, it is not unusual for an essentially psychogenic pain to develop at the same site that a lost parent had pain when alive.
6. Pain can also be associated with sexual feelings. At the height of sexual stimulation, pain may be mutually inflicted and enjoyed. When such activity assumes a dominant role in sexual activity, we label it perversion and sadomasochism.

The psychological meanings associated with pain are indeed complex and reflect the mixing of personal historical events, private meanings, untoward experiences with illness and pain, and the internalization of pains associated with parents or caregivers. It is this idiosyncratic meaning ascribed to pain by the patient that complicates the clinical picture. The majority of meanings that are subsumed within the individual psychic signature are unconscious. Because many of these idiosyncratic meanings have their origins in early trauma, they are often repressed, dissociated, or foreclosed from consciousness. Major painful illness or trauma has the capacity to loosen the moorings of these events in the unconscious, and the psychotherapist working with a chronic pain patient may find that after a therapeutic alliance has been established the patient finds him/herself bothered by a flooding of anxious dreams, terrifying images, or nameless dreads (Grzesiak, 1991c, 1992). Parenthetically, the majority of pain patients never engage in an uncovering type of psychotherapy, and it is important that health care personnel who engage in hands-on treatment (e.g., physicians, dentists, chiropractors, and physical therapists) develop some familiarity with and sensitivity to behaviors that signal the possibility of early trauma. An example would be the patient who becomes inexplicably anxious when being manipulated by the physical therapist or examined by the physician.

Engel provided us with two major papers that described his clinical findings in pain-prone patients (1951, 1959). Only recently have there appeared papers demonstrating these correlations from more controlled, although still retrospective, investigations. Only one of these studies will be reviewed here. In a retrospective controlled study, Adler and associates (1989) attempted to validate Engel's early developmental experiences across four groups of patients: (1) psychogenic pain, (2) organic pain, (3) psychogenic bodily symptoms, and (4) organic disease. The group of patients with psychogenic pain was found to be statistically significantly different from the other three groups with regard to the following factors: (1) parents who were verbally or physically abusive of each other, (2) parents who were abusive of the child, (3) children who deflected aggression from one parent to the other onto themselves, (4) parents who suffered from illness or painful conditions, (5) parent of same gender as the patient suffering from pain, (6) pain of patient and parent in the same location, (7) greater number of surgeries in adulthood, and (8) disturbed interpersonal relations and work life (Adler, Zlot, Hurny, & Minder, 1989). This study as well as others to be mentioned suggest that the onset, course, convalescence, and recovery from illness may be shaped by unconscious or preconscious factors that do not reside within the patient's awareness, yet profoundly affect the patient. The most profound effect is the capacity to embrace suffering.

A concept closely related to pain proneness is that of the dysthymic pain disorder (Blumer & Heilbronn, 1989). In fact, they speak of their work as a validation and extension of Engel's concept of pain proneness. On the basis of extensive clinical work with pain patients, Blumer and Heilbronn (1989) believe that pain in the absence of demonstrable physical findings reflects an underlying depression. Patients with dysthymic pain disorder have very characteristic histories. Their personality is a presentation of hypernormalcy; they deny psychological and interpersonal difficulties, present as the epitome of responsibility both familially and vocationally, and are pathologically self-reliant. They have a history of excessive work performance, frequently hold more than one job, are uncomfortable with time off, rarely take vacations, and do little in the way of relaxation. Typically, they have maintained this pace from early in life, often having been forced to enter the work force precociously to provide for family members in the face of the parents' failure to do so. When these individuals suffer an accident, illness, or trauma resulting in pain, they initially have extreme difficulty in allowing themselves to be ill but finally succumb to their dependency needs to such an extent that recovery and rehabilitation become problematic. Blumer and Heilbronn have found the developmental histories of these patients filled with conflict, abuse, and abandonment. All these experiences are inputs in one's psychological self/body self via the individual psychic signature and contribute to an identity or "sense of self" that embraces suffering.

The Neural Signature

Earlier, I spoke of Engel's "pain memories" or "body pain image" as having the capacity to complicate adult clinical pain. At this point, I would like to expand on this idea using the work of Melzack (1989, 1991, 1992). In a review article, Melzack and Loeser (1978) proposed a central "pattern generating mechanism" as being responsible for pain perception in the absence of afferent input in paraplegics. Disruption of the central nervous system (as is found in paraplegia where there is complete transection of the spinal cord) has profound implications for both excitatory and inhibitory mechanisms within the nervous system. Because many paraplegics experience pain below the level of their spinal lesion, Melzack & Loeser (1978) argue for two conclusions: (1) the mechanisms that underlie these pains must be sought central to the level of cord transection, and (2) the loss of input to central structures after deafferentation may play an important role in producing pain. Simply put, it is the loss of input to brain areas subserving pain that leads to nerve impulses exceeding threshold levels with resulting pain experience. Thus, a central pattern generating mechanism is established that leads to the experience of pain in the lost or nonfunctional body part. Once this central pattern generating mechanism is established, it may run autonomously for indefinite periods. Additionally, it may be triggered by a variety of stimuli, including psychological ones (Melzack & Loeser, 1978). Just as excitatory patterns can be triggered by psychological factors, so too can inhibitory or modulating effects be imparted to the central pattern generating mechanism by psychological input. In a clinical report, I demonstrated the successful, long-term reduction of pain in three out of four paraplegic patients by teaching them a simple relaxation paradigm (Grzesiak, 1977).

Based on both laboratory and clinical work, Melzack has expanded the concept of a central pattern generating mechanism and developed a much more complex theory of the "body pain image" (1989, 1991, 1992). Using phantom-limb pain as the most applicable human model, Melzack (1989) has proposed his concept of the "neuromatrix" (Fig. 1.1). According to Melzack: "It is proposed that we are born with a widespread neural network—the neuromatrix—for the body self, which is subsequently modified by experience. The neuromatrix imparts a pattern—the neurosignature—on

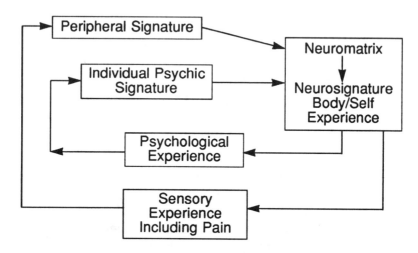

FIGURE 1.1   Neuromatrix.

all inputs from the body, so that experiences of one's own body have a quality of self and are imbued with affective tone and cognitive meaning" (p. 208). Again, according to Melzack (1991): "The anatomical substrate of the body self . . . is a large, widespread network of neurons that consists of loops between the thalamus and cortex as well as between the cortex and limbic system" (1991, p. 61). In support of the concept of a neuromatrix, Melzack offered the following four propositions, along with supporting clinical and experimental evidence.

> Proposition 1. "The experience of a phantom limb has the quality of reality because it is produced by the same brain processes that underlie the experience of the body when it is intact" (1989, p. 208).
> Proposition 2. "Neural networks in the brain generate all the qualities of experience that are felt to originate in the body; inputs from the body may trigger or modulate the output of the networks but are not essential for any of the qualities of experience" (1989, p. 209).
> Proposition 3. "The experience of the body has a unitary integrated quality that includes the quality of the "self"—

that the body is uniquely one's own and not that of any
other individual" (1989, p. 209).
Proposition 4. "The neural network that underlies the experience of the body–self is genetically determined but
can be modified by sensory experience" (1989, p. 209).

While Melzack has used phantom limb pain as his model of
choice, he does provide us with examples from other deafferentation injuries and surgical procedures as well. In one of his most recent papers, he was somewhat less optimistic about the capacity of
new sensory experiences to modify pain sensation (Melzack, 1992).
However, the implications of the neuromatrix extend far beyond
pain management; Melzack is clear that the neuromatrix holds
"experience, affect, and meaning" (1991, p. 62). Those are clearly
dimensions of psychological functioning and I would suggest that
the neuromatrix contains our identity; not only body-self but psychological self as well. Further, following from that, I would suggest that psychological experience, which includes sensory experience, has the capacity to modify the neuromatrix as well.

Combining the Peripheral, Psychic, and Neural Signatures

Although it is common knowledge that persistent pain undergoes a
centralization process through which it can become independent of
its peripheral origins, what are the implictions for understanding
mind–body interaction as it relates to pain and suffering? If one
combines Melzack's concept of the neuromatrix with Engel's concept of pain proneness, then the neural signature would actually
hold both the peripheral and the individual psychic signatures.
Perhaps we could then conceive of a psychoneurobiology that had
greater explanatory power regarding how experience can modify
sensation. In recent years, there have been a number of scholarly
efforts to combine mind and body (e.g., Reiser, 1983; Rossi, 1986).
Reiser, for example, searched for explanations enabling a convergence of the psychoanalytic model of mind with its neurobiologic
underpinnings (Reiser, 1983). In doing so, he drew heavily on memory research, including the work by Kandel (1978) demonstrating
that there is memory at the cellular level. Reiser asked, just what
are the processes that enable a transformation of psychic experience into brain response and can it be reprogrammed? If informa-

tion, be it sensory or psychic, is given the same valence, perhaps we can move a step closer to understanding that psychogenic pain and somatogenic pain are merely different sides of the same coin. In an articulate attempt to explain the nature of mind–body healing, Rossi (1986) concluded that the only common denominator extending from cellular level to cognition, and encompassing virtually all organ systems, was information. Can experience modify neural systems? Clearly it can, but what are the implications for pain management? What does this add to our understanding of the nature of vulnerability to chronic suffering?

Two recent studies, one a retrospective review and the other a clinical case report, suggest that when there are experiences in the person's background that relate to suffering or pain proneness, the appropriate medical or surgical treatment may not lead to pain relief. In an attempt to determine whether or not early developmental experiences could have an impact on the outcome of spinal surgery, Schofferman and associates operationalized Engel's developmental events into five sets of risk factors (Schofferman, Anderson, Hines, et al., 1992). The risk factors were as follows: (1) physical abuse by a parent or primary caregiver, (2) emotional abuse by a parent or primary caregiver, (3) sexual abuse by a primary caregiver or other adult, (4) abandonment or loss of a primry caregiver during childhood or adolescence, and (5) parents or caregivers who were either alcoholic or otherwise substance abusors. They correlated the presence or absence of these risk factors with the outcome of spinal surgery in patients who were clearly in need of such surgery. The evaluators were blind to surgical outcome and convalescence at the time they reviewed the charts and psychiatric reports for risk factors. They found that for those patients who remembered none of the risk factors as having happened to them during their formative years, the successful postsurgical outcome, convalescence and return to previous level of functioning was 95%. For those patients who remembered three or more of the risk factors as having been part of their personal history, the successful outcome dropped to 15%. The relationship was linear, with the presence of each risk factor adding to the probability of poor outcome. Now, what happened here? The appropriate surgery was done for an identified pathology but yet in those patients at risk, outcome was poor. This is a somewhat frightening finding because it suggests that for patients who have a vulnerability to suffering, a matrix of psychodevelopmental events laying an unconscious foundation for pain proneness, the appropriate procedure may not work. Schofferman et al. chose to make their primary explanation a relational one and used attachment theory to describe how the early trauma had made it difficult, if not impossible, for these patients to allow themselves to be sick and taken care of, therefore confounding their own recoveries (see Chapter 6). This appears to be a reasonable explanation because object relations theory in psychoanalysis does allow for one's relationship with one's self (and, I would add, body self) as well as with others. But what if the input to the neuromatrix is an unconsciously driven psychic signature that embraces pain and suffering? The peripheral problem has been eliminated, but the psychic signature requiring pain and suffering has been fused with earlier peripheral signatures into a central pattern generating mechanism that essentially defines body-self as "painful self." If this is in fact the case, then in addition to those pharmacologic agents used to alter central mechanisms, one certainly would need to consider psychotherapy as well, probably intensive long-term psychotherapy, because these problems in coming to terms with persistent pain do not reflect focal difficulties or coping failure but rather reflect matters of identity and character (Grzesiak, 1991c, 1992).

Is it necessary for the trauma to occur at developmentally early points in time for there to be a psychic signature requiring suffering? Apparently not. Harness and Donlon (1988) presented two cases of intractable facial pain in which abuse in adulthood led to symptoms unresponsive to treatment for years. It was only when the patients established a solid therapeutic alliance and trusted their therapists that they were able to reveal the actual origins of their pain, namely, physical abuse. In both cases they had hidden the abuse from their doctors for years. I would speculate that because the origins of their pains were physically traumatic, the peripheral afferent input (signature) fused with a dissociated psychic signature and spilled both into the neuromatrix. The experience of trauma, be it severe physical or sexual abuse, is usually processed by the mind in a state-dependent or dissociated state so that it is not in storage where ordinary recall can retrieve it.

What I am suggesting is a profoundly central theory of pain and suffering in which both body-self experience and psychological self experience mesh and are held in place within the neuromatrix.

One of the major implications of this particular view is that both sensory and psychological experience have the same valence; either one is capable of altering the ongoing neural signature and affecting body self and psychological self.

Implications for Chronic Pain Syndromes

When one considers the many permutations that are possible between the peripheral signature and the individual psychic signature, it seems probable that many chronic pain syndromes have a significant psychological component, although that component may or may not involve psychological conflict. Because most of the clinical and theoretical examples used in this chapter thus far have involved back pain, I want to use chronic orofacial pain as a way of illustrating some of the concepts defined above involving the integration of peripheral, psychic, and neural signatures. So often in the orofacial pain clinic we see individuals who have developed intractable or persistent pain in the oral cavity or facial area following dental procedures. Technically, the dental work looks good. Why does the pain persist? Is it psychogenic? Probably not in the usual sense of the word "psychogenic." The concept of the neuromatrix enables us to make sense of these orofacial pain conditions, often thought to be of unknown origin or related to deafferentation.

The oral cavity is one of the most personally sensitive areas of our body self. We know from Freud and his followers that the first stage of psychosexual development is the oral one with all its implications, ranging from passive receptivity to aggression. The face and oral cavity are also imbued with a profound body narcissism; it is how we meet the world, take in the world, and let the world see us. Changes in the oral cavity or related facial musculature are usually experienced in augmented or exaggerated sensation. As one recent patient said to me about her bite: "A millimeter feels like a mile." Changes in dentition, microtrauma to related neural structures, adaptation to implants, and new bridges all feed new and different sensory input through the peripheral signature to the neuromatrix. Because facial areas also represent a heavily invested sense of both psychological self and body self, any differences in peripheral signature are likely to trigger private meanings that are then input through the individual psychic signature to the neuromatrix as well. Many of the chronic orofacial pain conditions involve older patients, and one could speculate on how changes in the neural pool that Melzack assumes comprise the neuromatrix lose their plasticity. Consequently, new information fed into the neuromatrix by both peripheral and psychic signatures may not be accommodated. From a psychological perspective, such lack of accommodation between peripheral signature, individual psychic signature, and what the neuromatrix will accept in terms of neural modification may lead to some of the more frequently observed symptoms in chronic pain patients; for example, somatic preoccupation, somatization, and depression.

Summary

This review of some of the more common biopsychosocial components of vulnerability is based primarily on clinical experience. In presenting a biopsychosocial model of symptom formation, it was my goal to provide the reader with a flavor for how a wide variety of risk factors can serve as predisposers, triggers, and buffers for stress-related symptoms, including pain. This is not meant to imply that all pain, including chronic pain syndrome, is related to stress, for that simply is not so. The role of psychological factors in the development of chronic pain varies greatly and may include learning, coping failure, deficits in coping skills, vocational dissatisfaction, psychological illness, and psychiatric problems. Clinical experience with chronic pain patients, particularly those who develop chronic pain syndromes, has led to a greater appreciation of the role of developmental factors, particularly trauma and abuse, in forming a vulnerability to pain proneness. The empirical literature on the role of trauma in the development of chronic pain syndromes is sketchy at best. However, it is important to reiterate that the experience of trauma, abuse, or abandonment early in life is rarely clearly remembered since it is most appropriate for defensive operations such as repression and dissociation to protect the self from such awareness. Recollections of early trauma, may only appear in the face of new trauma and then both current and historical events complicate the clinical picture.

The matrix of vulnerability refers to the hidden, usually unconscious, foundation for pain proneness that is a consequence of psychosocial/developmental experiences that involve illness, pain, aggression, guilt, and suffering. I have taken liberties with Melzack's concept of the central pattern generating mechanism and its advanced formulation as the neuromatrix to demonstrate how this vulnerability to suffering can be embedded within the neural pool waiting to be activated by illness or trauma. Within this framework, I propose that psychological self and body self have equal valence and are both a part of the neural signature from the neuromatrix. Implicit in this formulation is the idea that both psychological experience and sensory experience define one's sense of self, both in health and in illness. Within this framework, one can more easily understand how psychotherapy and other psychological interventions can alter adaptation to persistent pain and potentially reverse or prevent the development of chronic pain syndromes.

References

Adler, R. H., Zlot, S., Horny, C., & Minder, C. (1989). Engel's "Psychogenic pain and the pain-prone patient." A retrospective controlled clinical study. *Psychosomatic Medicine, 51,* 87–101.

Barber, T. X. (1969). *Hypnosis: A scientific approach.* New York: Van Nostrand Reinhold.

Blumer, D., & Heilbronn, M. (1989). Dysthmyic pain disorder: The treatment of chronic pain as a variant of depression. In C. D. Tollison (Ed.), *Handbook of chronic pain management* (pp. 197–209). Baltimore: Williams & Wilkins.

Ciccone, D. S., & Grzesiak, R. C. (1984). Cognitive dimensions of chronic pain. *Social Science & Medicine,* 19, 1339–1345.

Ciccone, D. S., & Grzesiak, R. C. (1990). Chronic musculoskeletal pain: A cognitive approach to psychophysiologic assessment and intervention. In M. G. Eisenberg, & R. C. Grzesiak (Eds.), *Advances in clinical rehabilitation, vol. 3* (pp. 197–214). New York: Springer Publishing Co.

Crue, B. L. Jr. (1978). *Evaluation of chronic pain syndromes. (tape T155).* New York: BioMonitoring Applications.

DeLongis, A., Coyne, J. C., Dakof, G., et al. (1982). Relationship of daily hassles, uplifts and major life events to health status. *Health Psychology, 1,* 119–136.

Diagnostic and statistical manual of mental disorders, revised, 3rd Edition. (1987). Washington, DC: American Psychiatric Association.

Dworkin, R. H., & Grzesiak, R. C. (1993). Chronic pain: On the integration of psyche and soma. In G. Stricker & J. R. Gold (Eds.), *Comprehensive handbook of psychotherapy integration* (pp. 365–384). New York: Plenum.

Dworkin, R. H., Hartstein, G., Rosner, H. L., et al. (1992). A high-risk method for studying psychosocial antecedents of chronic pain: The prospective investigation of herpes zoster. *Journal of Abnormal Psychology, 101,* 200–205.

Dworkin, S. F., Von Korff, M., & LeResche, L. (1990). Multiple pains and psychiatric disturbance: An epidemiologic investigation. *Archives of General Psychiatry, 47,* 239–244.

Ellis, A. A. (1962). *Reason and emotion in psychotherapy.* New York: Lyle Stuart.

Engel, G. L. (1951). Primary atypical facial neuralgia: An hysterical conversion symptom. *Psychosomatic Medicine, 13,* 375–396.

Engel, G. L. (1959). "Psychogenic" pain and the pain-prone patient. *American Journal of Medicine, 26,* 899–918.

Eysenck, H. J. (1983). Psychophysiology and personality. In A. False & J. A. Edward (Eds.), *Physiological correlates of human behavior* (pp. 13–30). London: Academic.

Fordyce, W. E. (1976). *Behavioral methods for chronic pain and illness.* St. Louis: Mosby.

Freud, S. (1905). A fragment of an analysis of a case of hysteria. *Collected papers, vol. 3* (pp. 13–145). New York: Basic Books.

Freud, S., & Breuer, J. (1895/1955). Studies on hysteria. *Standard edition, vol. 2.* (pp. 1–305). London: Hogarth Press.

Grzesiak, R. C. (1977). Relaxation techniques in treatment of chronic pain. *Archives of Physical Medicine and Rehabilitation, 58,* 270–272.

Grzesiak, R. C. (1988). Psychologic aspects of chronic orofacial pain. I. Psychologic mechanisms. *Compendium of Continuing Education in Dentistry, 9,* 222–229.

Grzesiak, R. C. (1991a). Psychologic considerations in temporomandibular dysfunction: A biopsychosocial view of symptom formation. *Dental Clinics of North America, 35,* 209–226.

Grzesiak, R. C. (1991b). Psychological aspects of chronic orofacial pain: Theory, assessment and management. *Pain Digest, 1,* 100–119.

Grzesiak, R. C. (1991c, March). *Toward a psychotherapy for the chronic pain patient: Some directions.* Paper presented at the Annual Meeting of the Society of Behavioral Medicine. Washington, DC.

Grzesiak, R. C. (1992, August). *Unconscious processes and chronic pain: On the foundations of pain-proneness.* Paper presented at the Annual Meeting of the American Psychological Association. Washington, DC.

Harness, D. M., & Donlon, W. C. (1988). Cryptotrauma: The hidden wound. *Clinical Journal of Pain, 4,* 257–260.

Holmes, T. H., & Rahe, R. H. (1967). The social readjustment rating scale. *Journal of Psychosomatic Research, 11,* 213–218.

Kandel, E. R. (1978). *A Cell Biological Approach to Learning.* Bethesda: Society for Neuroscience.

Kanner, A. D., Coyne, J. C., Schaefer, C., et al. (1981). Comparison of two modes of stress measurement: Daily hassles and uplifts versus major life events. *Journal of Behavioral Medicine, 4,* 1–39.

Lacey, J. I. (1967). Somatic response patterning and stress: Some revisions of activation theory. In M. H. Appley & R. Trumball (Eds.), *Psychological stress.* pp. 14–42). New York: Appleton-Century-Crofts.

Lazarus, R. S., & Folkman, S. (1984). *Stress, appraisal and coping.* New York: Springer Publishing Co.

Loeser, J. D. (1982). Concepts of pain. In M. Stanton-Hicks & R. A. Boas (Eds.), *Chronic low back pain.* (pp. 145–148). New York: Raven.

Loeser, J. D., & Black, R. (1975). A taxonomy of pain. *Pain, 1,* 81–90.

Melzack, R. (1989). Phantom limbs. *Regional Anesthesia, 14,* 208–211.

Melzack, R. (1991). Central pain syndromes and theories of pain. In K. L. Casey (Ed.), *Pain and central nervous system disease: The central pain syndromes* (pp. 59–64). New York: Raven.

Melzack, R. (1992, April). Phantom limbs. *Scientific American,* 120–126.

Melzack, R., & Loeser, J. D. (1978). Phantom body pain in paraplegics: Evidence for a central "pattern generating mechanism" for pain. *Pain, 4,* 195–210.

Merskey, H. (1986). Classification of chronic pain: Descriptions of chronic pain syndromes and definitions of pain terms. *Pain,* Suppl. 3.

Middaugh, S. J., & Kee, W. G. (1987). Advances in electromyographic monitoring and biofeedback in the treatment of chronic cervical and low back pain. In M. G. Eisenberg & R. C. Grzesiak (Eds.), *Advances in clinical rehabilitation, vol. 1* (pp. 137–172). New York: Springer Publishing Co.

Pennebaker, J. W, (1985). Traumatic experience and psychosomatic disease: Exploring the roles of behavioral intervention, obsession, and confiding. *Canadian Psychologist, 26,* 82–95.

Reiser, M. F. (1983). *Mind, brain, body: Toward a convergence of psychoanalysis and neurobiology.* New York: Basic Books.

Rossi, E. L. (1986). *The psychobiology of mind–body healing: New concepts of therapeutic hypnosis.* New York: Norton.

Rudy, T. E., Turk, D. C., Zaki, H. S., & Curtin, H. D. (1989). An empirical taxometric alternative to traditional classification of temporomandibular disorders. *Pain, 36,* 311–320.

Schofferman, J., Anderson, D., Hines, R., Smith, G., & White, A. (1992). Childhood psychological trauma correlates with unsuccessful lumbar spine surgery. *Spine, 17*(Suppl), S138–144.

Sternbach, R. A. (1966) *Principles of psychophysiology.* New York: Academic.

Tait, R. C. (1983). Psychological factors in chronic benign pain. *Current concepts of pain, 1,* 10–15.

Turk, D. C., & Rudy, T. E. (1988). Toward an empirically derived taxonomy of chronic pain patients: Integration of psychological assessment data. *Journal of Consulting and Clinical Psychology, 56*, 233–238.

Turk, D. C., & Rudy, T. E. (1990). Neglected factors in chronic pain treatment outcome studies—referral patterns, failure to enter treatment, and attrition. *Pain, 43*, 7–25.

Turk, D. C., & Rudy, T. E. (1991). Neglected topics in the treatment of chronic pain patients—relapse, noncompliance, and adherence enhancement. *Pain, 44*, 5–28.

van der Kolk, B. A. (1989). The compulsion to repeat the trauma: Re-enactment, revictimization, and masochism. *Psychiatric Clinics of North America, 12*, 389–409.

van der Kolk, B. A., & van der Hart, O. (1991). The intrusive past: The flexibility of memory and the engraving of trauma. *American Imago, 48*, 425–454.

Wickramasekera, I. (1986). A model of people at high risk to develop chronic stress-related somatic symptoms: Some predictions. *Professional Psychology, 17*, 437–447.

Chapter Two

Somatizing as a Risk Factor for Chronic Pain

Samuel F. Dworkin, Leanne Wilson, and Donna L. Massoth

Introduction and Rationale

A common occurrence in primary medical care is the presentation of physical symptoms, most frequently pain, for which there is: (a) no readily apparent cause and no physical diagnosis can be discerned; (b) symptom complaint that is not commensurate with physical pathology, if present; (c) denial of psychological illness; and/or (d) psychological distress accompanying the physical complaints that is apparent as some measurable form of anxiety or depression (Goldberg & Huxley, 1992). Whether fairly or not, such patients are viewed as *somatizers* and the process they manifest is labeled *somatization*.

In this chapter we examine the relationship between the symptom of self-reported chronic pain and the process of somatization, specifically exploring the conditions under which somatization may constitute a risk factor—that is, may be associated with increased vulnerability—for the onset and maintenance of chronic pain conditions. A model developed earlier (Dworkin, Von Korff, & LeResche, 1992) is used to guide our discussion of somatization as a risk factor for chronic pain. The concept of somatization is elaborated from alternative theoretical perspectives, and attempts are made to distinguish somatization from overlapping and equally complex notions such as hypochondriasis and the related formal psychiatric somatoform diagnoses of Somatization Disorder and Somatoform Pain Disorder. Following this overview of somatization, and within the context of the model provided, we examine evidence that somatization is associated with increased risk of developing a pain condition; increased risk for duration or diffuseness of pain, or for pain-related disability; increased risk for poor treatment outcome; and increased risk for high health care utilization or excessive, potentially iatrogenic, medical treatment. We also address how anxiety and depression are related to the interaction between pain and somatization. For the most part, we focus on orofacial pain conditions in this discussion, both because we have ample research and clinical data in this area and because this condition shares many features with other more prevalent chronic pain conditions, such as back pain and headache (Von Korff, Dworkin, LeResche, & Kruger, 1988).

A Biopsychosocial Model for Chronic Pain: An Overview

Chronic pain is most usefully understood within the broader context of illness behavior, for as Eisenberg (1986) has pointed out:

> What brings patients to doctors is discomfort and dysfunction, not the pathology which underlies them. It matters—and matters greatly—to strategies for cure just how far bodily malfunction is causing problems of living and how far symptoms are the somatic embodiment of problems in living . . . in this process biomedical knowledge is necessary but not sufficient; the doctor's transactions with the patient must be informed by the social sciences. (p. 505)

As is abundantly evident through this book, it is well accepted that chronic pain arises from multiple and interrelated biologic, psychologic and social factors. The rich diversity of expression observed in the presentation of chronic pain results from the complex ways in which physical changes can be detected and appraised under the influence of social and cultural forces that shape acceptable manifestations of the sick role in any given society. The ecologic model of chronic pain we have developed (Dworkin, Von Korff, & LeResche, 1992) to guide our own thinking, clinical activity and research, draws on the work of Loeser (1980), Melzack and Wall (1965), Fordyce (1976), Mechanic (1986), Parsons (1975), and others (Kleinman, 1988; Pilowsky, Spence, Cobb, & Katsikitis, 1984; Turk & Flor, 1987) and has been put forth to describe these interactions. The model is consistent with our current biopsychosocial understanding of illness, and when the model is applied to chronic pain, it assumes noxious or nociceptive signals arising from changing physiologic states. These physiologic signals recruit higher order central processes of perception, appraisal, emotional arousal, and, eventually, pain behavior. Perceptual processes identify the noxious stimulus as painful in terms of its physical qualities, yielding such determinations as pain that is dull or sharp, mild or severe, well-localized or diffuse, and brief or long-lasting. The perception of pain leads to a cognitive-emotional appraisal process in which the individual assigns personal meaning to the pain—for example, does the pain signal serious illness, is it frightening or nonthreatening, does it require medical treatment? The appraisal process yields simultaneous emotional arousal that further reinforces the meaning ascribed to the painful event or condition.

These processes—nociception, perception, and appraisal—occur within the individual (i.e., are intrapersonal), and may eventually lead to observable (i.e., overt) pain behaviors that have an important interpersonal and social function—they communicate to others something of the suffering being experienced and reveal coping methods undertaken to address the pain. Finally, these chronic pain behaviors are understood to take place within the context of socially defined norms for the sick role—the chronic-pain patient is relieved of responsibilities at home, work, or school and is allowed to withdraw socially. Simultaneously, other chronic pain behaviors sanctioned by the socially defined sick role may increase, principally heightened reliance on health-care delivery in the form of increased medical visits, diagnostic tests, hospitalization, surgery, and the use of medications.

Goldberg (Goldberg & Huxley, 1992) has persuasively argued that common mental disorders, which include the highly prevalent manifestations of anxiety (including panic conditions) and depression, represent a continuum of nonspecific distress in the population and are to be distinguished from more severe, but fortunately rarer, conditions of severe mental illness, such as schizophrenia, organic brain syndromes, and bipolar affective disorders. Similarly, numerous others, including Katon (Katon et al., 1991), Kleinman (1988), and Escobar (Escobar et al., 1987), have argued that somatization is a common problem, reflecting the physical, affective, and behavioral status of large numbers of patients in primary medical care, while Somatoform Disorders as defined by the *Diagnostic and Statistical Manual of Mental Disorders* (DSM-III-R) (American Psychiatric Association, 1987) are, in fact, much rarer psychiatric disorders, seen most frequently only in specialized tertiary care facilities. Escobar, Burnam, Karno, Forsythe, and Golding (1987) and Escobar et al. (1987) have defined so-called subsyndromal forms of somatization (subsyndromal because they do not meet the rigid criteria for large numbers of physical symptoms required to diagnose Somatization Disorder according to DSM-III-R). The prevalence of these subsyndromal disorders in the population varies from 4% to 12%, compared to a prevalence for Somatization Disorder of less than 1%. Katon (Katon et al., 1991) has introduced the notion of somatization as a process with a *spectrum of severity*, rather than a psychiatric condition that is dichotomously absent or present. Subsyndromal forms of Somatization Disorder, typically seen in primary care, are consistently found to be significantly associated with higher rates of medical utilization, disability, and the relatively common symptoms of anxiety and depression as well as higher rates for lifetime diagnoses of Dysthymic Disorder and Major Depressive Disorder.

Simon (1991) has distinguished among four levels for analyzing somatization as a concept engaging the presence of poorly understood physical symptoms. At the perceptual level, somatization represents a *nonspecific amplification of distress* such that aversive psychologic states lead to increased arousal and vigilance that are inevitably associated with lowered threshold for perceiving and reporting bodily events (Barsky, 1979; Barsky, Goodson, Lane, et al., 1988). Selective focus on noxious sensations can become a pathway for the channeling of nonspecific distress to physical symptoms.

Somatization as a *psychological defense* involves appraisal-emotional factors and is exemplified by the view of chronic pain as a "masked" depression (Blumer & Heilbronn, 1982). According to this view, pain is experienced and expressed instead of depression—that is, the presence of a chronic pain condition serves the psychological defense of masking depression. The notion of somatization as an idiom of expression of psychological distress (Katon et al.,

1991; Kleinman, 1988) is also relevant here, reflecting that physical symptoms are appraised as indicative of physical pathology while denying psychological disturbance.

The third level, that of somatization as a *tendency to seek care* for common symptoms (Mechanic, 1986), incorporates illness behavior into the concept of somatization. According to this view, somatizers adopt learned patterns of coping with emotional distress that result in a focus on bodily symptoms leading to excessive health-care utilization. Such learned patterns are often culturally sanctioned and reinforced, particularly in Western cultures where society has become highly "medicalized."

Finally, the concept of somatization as a *consequence of health care utilization* (i.e., due to the tendency of cultural factors and medical providers to reinforce presentation of physical symptoms) places a component of responsibility for inappropriate pain-related illness behavior on the health-care delivery system and other social institutions that selectively attend to physical symptoms at the expense of accompanying psychological distress. This environmental reinforcement, through "over-medicalization" of the patient's symptom presentation, may potentially contribute to iatrogenic somatization.

An important additional step in defining somatization is clarifying the distinction between somatization and hypochondriasis. The concepts are overlapping; both are characterized by a focus on physical symptoms and function. The central feature of hypochondriasis is a cognitive appraisal process revealing a preoccupation with the fear of having, or the belief one has, a serious disease. Hypochondriacal thinking is often associated with health care behaviors that appear obsessive and that are barely responsive to reassurance. Hypochondriacal behavior tends to engage a very specific or focal symptom, while somatization tends to involve numerous symptoms or shifts in symptomatology from one area of the body to another over time. Illness behaviors such as excessive limitations of daily activities or inappropriate health-care seeking are a frequent, although not inevitable, consequence of both hypochondriasis and somatization.

The major link that connects the theoretical perspectives of somatization offered above with the clinical realities of engaging the chronic pain patient resides in the patient's explanatory model for their pain and physical symptoms in general. Explanatory models of illness are defined by Kleinman (1988) as the "notions that patients, families and practitioners have about a specific illness episode." Explanatory models represent an attempt by the individual to make sense of the illness experience—that is, how one perceives, experiences, and copes with illness. Each individual carries a set of illness beliefs about the etiology of their illness, the time and mode of onset of symptoms, what maintains or aggravates their symptoms, and the expected course of their illness and appropriate treatments. These beliefs and expectancies are shaped by past illness episodes as they are personally experienced or observed in others. Once an individual notices symptoms, a process of retrospectively linking symptoms with beliefs from the illness repertoire occurs (Chrisman, 1977). The explanatory models which emerge can be simple, obscure, complex, or precise. Importantly, these models of illness beliefs are specific to the individual and are influenced by ethnocultural variables governing perception, labeling, explanation, and valuation of the illness experience. Thus, the processes that interact in chronic pain and illness are embedded in a complex family, social, and cultural nexus (Litman, 1974).

We ascribe critical saliency to the patient's explanatory model for two reasons. First, the patient's explanatory model serves to organize their perceptions, motivations, and behavior with regard to what they will or will not do about their chronic pain. In addition, a major therapeutic objective usually required for chronic pain patients is to modify their presenting explanatory model away from its typically preeminent physical focus, which also carries the expectation that factors in the environment—for example, doctors—hold the "cure" to their condition. Biobehavioral interventions that emphasize increased reliance on self-care and the assumption of greater self-responsibility for effective coping with pain are needed to redirect or otherwise modify the chronic-pain patient's well-learned, albeit usually unrealistic, expectations of care providers.

In summary, these views collectively suggest that somatization may be most usefully understood as a dimension of personal functioning characterized by the tendency to report distress arising from perceived physical symptoms that typically are not consistent with measurable physiologic or pathophysiologic changes. This tendency can vary in its intensity among individuals, including among pain patients, and can also fluctuate within an individual across situations and the lifespan. It is particularly important to emphasize that, in our view, the concept of somatization comprises two domains: (1) a perceptual–cognitive predisposition to evaluate perceived physical signals as symptoms of a problem in the body, and (2) the behavioral predisposition towards symptom-reporting and treatment-seeking. Thus, the predisposition to focus perceptually and cognitively on physical symptoms is not only associated with apparent insensitivity to accompanying psychological distress but also with a subset of maladaptive illness behaviors. Such behaviors, characterized by Fordyce (1976) as *chronic pain behaviors*, include severe limitations in meeting social responsibilities and excessive use of health care in pursuit of a cure for a physical problem. This maladaptive pattern of coping with chronic pain, previously labeled *chronic pain syndrome*, has more recently been called *dysfunctional chronic pain*. That researchers and clinicians in the area assume conceptual overlap between dysfunctional chronic pain and somatization is supported by the inclusion of Somatoform Pain Disorder as one of the Somatoform Disorders in the DSM-III-R (American Psychiatric Association, 1987). Further, studies have found a cross-sectional association between somatization and pain: individuals with chronic pain are likely to have elevated scores on measures of somatization (Dworkin, LeResche, & Von Korff, 1989). What is the evidence, however, that somatization is a *risk factor* for chronic pain?

Somatization as a Risk Factor for Chronic Pain: A Selected Review of Recent Findings

A narrow epidemiologic definition of "risk" is "the likelihood that people who are without a disease, but exposed to certain factors ("risk factors"), will acquire the disease" (Fletcher, Fletcher, & Wagner, 1988, p. 91). Von Korff suggests that for chronic pain, risk factors are also those variables that control or predict the probability of transition to increasing pain-related morbidity, such as behavioral limitations, psychosocial disruption, and other manifestations of disability. These risk factors can be classified as *initiators* (factors that set in motion a causal process), *promoters* (factors that enhance or potentiate a causal process already initiated), and *detection factors* (factors that have no causal effect but that increase the likelihood of a case being identified) (Von Korff et al., 1992).

Much of the data on somatization as a risk factor for chronic pain presented here focuses on temporomandibular disorders (TMD), which are facial pain conditions characterized by pain in the temporomandibular region, often accompanied by clicking or grating sounds in the temporomandibular joint and deviations and limitations in opening the jaw (American Dental Association, 1983). TMD is a relatively common chronic pain condition, affecting approximately 12% of the adult population according to epidemiologic studies. Women more frequently than men seek care for TMD at ratios of more than 4 or 5:1 (Moss, Garrett, & Chiodo, 1982; Von Korff, Dworkin, LeResche, & Kruger, 1988). TMD patients are comparable to those with back pain, abdominal pain, chest pain, and headache in pain intensity, duration, and health care utilization, but not in extent of pain-related activity limitation (e.g., inability to work) (Von Korff, Dworkin, LeResche, & Kruger, 1988). Rudy and Turk (1989) have shown that TMD patients have psychologic profile patterns similar to headache and back pain patients. In this chapter, we examine the relationship between somatization and TMD pain with the understanding that findings are likely to be relevant to our understanding of chronic benign pain conditions in general.

For chronic TMD pain, several classes of variables have been studied as risk factors: (1) biologic factors such as malocclusion, traumatic injury to the temporomandibular joint, displacement of the articular disk, and osteoarthritic changes, as well as disease states such as rheumatoid arthritis; (2) behavioral factors such as parafunctional habits (clenching or grinding of teeth), postural habits and other pathogenic behaviors such as gum chewing; and (3) psychosocial factors such as psychological distress, the experience of numerous stressful life events, and somatization. The extent to which biologic and behavioral factors are associated with onset and maintenance of TMD pain conditions has been extensively discussed in the literature (Dworkin, Von Korff, & LeResche, 1990; Greene & Marbach, 1982) and is beyond the scope of this chapter.

Somatization and Multiple Pains

To begin to unravel the intertwined threads of somatization, chronic pain, and psychologic distress, we will first examine connections between somatization and the report of multiple pain conditions. Somatization, as we have defined it, is a tendency of the individual to report distress arising from numerous physical symptoms which are poorly associated with confirmable physical abnormality. Characteristically, physical symptoms are dispersed across multiple organ systems and include symptoms such as gastrointestinal nausea or upset, heart palpitations, faintness or dizziness, feelings of weakness or heaviness in limbs, headaches, and other pains. Examination of the SCL-90-R somatization scale (Derogatis, 1983), a 12-item self-report inventory of physical symptoms, reveals that five of the items are pain-related and seven are non–pain symptoms. Epidemiologic and survey research indicate that recurrent pain is by far the most common type of somatic symptom reported (Escobar et al., 1987; Ketterer & Buckholtz, 1989; Smith, Monson, & Ray, 1985; Swartz, Blazer, Woodbury, George, & Landerman, 1986). Among the community respondents ($n = 3132$) from the Los Angeles sample of the National Institute of Mental Health Epidemiological Catchment Area study (NIMH-ECA), four pain symptoms (headache, painful menstrual periods, chest pain, and abdominal pain) were among the eight most common somatic symptoms reported (Escobar et al., 1987). In the North Carolina sample of the NIMH-ECA, Swartz and his colleagues (Swartz, Blazer, Woodbury, George, & Landerman, 1986) reported on the subset of respondents ($n = 1,626$) who endorsed at least three somatization symptoms. Among the top ten symptoms reported by this group, five were pain-related: 31% reported headaches, 27% painful menstrual periods, 24% chest pain, 19% abdominal pain, and 16% arm or leg pain.

A unique aspect of pain is its potential to be experienced in almost every organ system across anatomic sites—that is, chronic pain can be located in the musculoskeletal, cardiovascular, gastrointestinal, and other organ systems. We have posed the possibility of a form of somatization "where the symptom report is limited to pain, as in somatoform pain disorder, but where multiple pain conditions are identified in diverse regions or organ systems of the body, as in Somatization Disorder" (Dworkin, Von Korff, & LeResche, 1990). Multiple pains, in other words, could be understood to represent an aspect of or manifestation of somatization, and to be similarly associated with psychiatric distress or disturbance.

We conducted an epidemiologic study of chronic pain in which respondents were asked about the presence in the past 6 months of each of five pain conditions—back pain, headache, abdominal pain, chest pain, and TMD pain. The survey respondents were 1,016 active enrollees of Group Health Cooperative of Puget Sound, a large Health Maintenance Organization. The results indicated that slightly over one-third of the individuals (36.5%) reported having none of the five pain conditions, one-third (34.1 %) reported having one pain, 20% had two pains, and 9% had three or more pain conditions in the past 6 months (Von Korff, Dworkin, LeResche, & Kruger, 1988).

In comparing number of pains to SCL somatization score, the pain items on the SCL scale were excluded to yield a somatization score based on report of bodily symptoms other than pain, and high somatization was defined as the top 15% of the sample (Dworkin, Von Korff, & LeResche, 1990). Respondents reporting pain in two body regions were almost ten times as likely as persons with no pain to fall into this heightened somatization group; those with three or more other pains were 13 times as likely to do so as the nonpain group. Similar analyses indicated that the probability for an algorithm diagnosis of major depression (based on response to SCL depression-scale items analogous to DSM-III-R criteria for Major Depressive Disorders) increased five-to-eight-fold for individuals with two or more pain conditions, as compared to those with no pain. Interestingly, individuals with one pain problem were no more likely to meet the criteria for depression than were those reporting no pain, and the association between multiple pains and somatization was stronger than that between multiple pains and depression. These results support the view that multiple chronic pain conditions may represent a channel for expression of somatization.

In other analyses, we also examined whether the presence of a pain condition at one point in time increased the risk for onset of each of the other chronic pain conditions 3 years later. We compared two groups: those that were pain-free at first assessment, and those that had one or more pain conditions. For all the pain conditions except chest pain, the 3-year onset rates were statistically higher among individuals with a pain condition at baseline than for pain-free individuals. Because of the established relationship between depression and pain (Romano & Turner, 1985), we examined whether SCL depression score predicted pain onset. Depression score was associated with increased risk of first onset of headache and chest pain but not with the other three conditions. In addition, the relationship found between presence of a pain condition and increased likelihood of onset of each of the other conditions 3 years later was maintained while controlling for depression score. It appears that individuals with at least one pain condition are considerably more likely than those without pain to develop pain at a different site over time.

Somatization and Pain Dispersion

The picture emerging from these data is that, among a community-based sample, pain is both predictive of the onset of other pain conditions and likely to coexist with the report of numerous nonpain symptoms and psychiatric distress, with increasingly strong relationships as the number of pain conditions increases.

Within a sample of individuals presenting for treatment of TMD pain identified as part of the epidemiologic study described earlier, a similarly strong relationship between heightened somatization (as measured by the SCL) and number of other pain conditions was observed ($r = .54$). Furthermore, we found that somatization score was related to a TMD pain condition that was widely dispersed throughout the orofacial region. Subjects reported on TMD pain dispersion by: (1) reporting the location of their pain using a pain drawing, and (2) identifying painful sites during a clinical examination involving palpation of the muscles of the face, neck, and mouth (20 extraoral sites and 8 intraoral sites; 4 additional sites typically not expected to elicit TMD-related palpation pain were included as "placebo" sites). Somatization score was positively associated both with number of pain drawing sites ($r = 0.31$) and with number of examination sites (extraoral sites, $r = 0.46$; intraoral sites, $r = 0.42$).

When subjects were divided into three groups based on somatization score, the relationship between these groups and number of painful examination sites was highly significant. For extraoral muscle sites, for example, the low somatization group identified a mean of 3.2 painful sites, and the high somatization group identified a mean of 8.2 (of a possible 20) painful sites. A significant difference in painful placebo sites by somatization grouping was also found: 44% of the high somatization group reported one or more painful placebo sites, while only 15% of the low somatization group did so (Wilson et al., in press).

Previous studies have found similar relationships between somatization and pain report among chronic pain patients, particularly on self-report measures of pain location and quality. Schwartz and DeGood (1984) rated the pain drawings of a mixed sample of pain patients for their appropriateness based on dermatomal distribution, degree of bodily involvement, and anatomic sensibility. They found that patients with pain drawings rated as inappropriate reported a significantly higher number of somatic symptoms. Similarly, Gil et al. (1990) reported that sickle-cell disease patients whose pain location drawings were inconsistent with the disease condition were more likely to have clinically significant somatization scores. In a study of a pain clinic sample of patients with chronic facial, back, or extremity pain, patients reporting more spatially distributed pain obtained higher scores on the general hypochondriasis and disease conviction scales of the Illness Behavior Questionnaire (Toomey, Gover, & Jones, 1983).

Somatization and Pain-Related Behavior

Somatization and Disability

We turn now to the issue of whether there is a relationship between heightened somatization and pain-related disability among individuals with a chronic pain condition. Pain patients, of course, exhibit a range of pain-related disability or dysfunction: some individuals report that pain interferes significantly in their lives and frequently keeps them from performing work and social responsibilities, while others describe themselves as coping with pain such that it interferes minimally or not at all. Von Korff et al. (1992) developed a classification scheme for grading chronic pain disability. The classification scheme is based on self-report of pain intensity, pain-related disability days, and the extent to which pain interfered with work, recreational/social, and family activities. Patients with Grade 1 pain are those with low intensity, nondisabling pain; they report that pain interferes minimally with their usual activities. Grade 2 reflects high intensity but nondisabling pain. Grades

3 and 4 represent those individuals with moderate and severe pain dysfunction, and high intensity pain is typical of these patients. These patients report that to either a moderate or severe extent, pain is interfering with their ability to perform work and other social roles.

The graded pain classification system does not include somatization score as one of its criteria, and we would hypothesize that pain patients with more somatic symptoms are also more likely to be classified with a higher grade of pain-related disability. Our data confirm that pain grade and somatization score are significantly correlated among a sample of TMD patients ($r = 0.40$). The mean SCL somatization score for the Grade 1 patients was 0.56, compared with a mean somatization score of 1.10 for Grades 3 and 4 patients combined. In addition to being highly statistically significant, this difference is clinically meaningful: the somatization scores of the Grade 3 and 4 patients place them in the top 10% of a normal distribution for somatization score (Von Korff, Dworkin, LeResche, & Kruger, 1988), and indicate that they are endorsing a good deal of physical symptomatology. These data confirm that individuals with both a pain condition and high somatization score are also likely to report that their pain condition is having a negative impact on their lives.

Somatization and Treatment

As we have described, the two main dimensions incorporated into most definitions of somatization are the reporting of numerous somatic symptoms and the tendency to seek health care frequently. Yet, there are few data regarding the link between these two dimensions, either in general or among chronic pain patients. We have data from a sample of 190 individuals seeking treatment for their TMD that indicate that the number of self-reported somatic symptoms is related to treatment-seeking for chronic pain. Score on the SCL somatization scale was significantly correlated both with number of providers from whom the patients had sought treatment ($r = 0.33$) and with number of treatments received ($r = 0.26$). Although these correlations are modest, they suggest that individuals who are highly somatically focused also behave in a way that places them at increased risk for iatrogenic effects of health care—they seek multiple treatments from multiple providers. This point is made even more clearly by comparing the treatment seeking of those with somatization scores in the top 15% with those in the bottom 15%. We found that the mean number of providers seen by those with elevated scores was 6.9, compared with 2.2 providers for the low somatization group. The high somatization patients reported having received a mean of 4.4 different TMD pain treatments, while the mean for the low somatization group was 1.9.

It has also been hypothesized that a tendency to be somatically focused may be predictive of poor response to pain treatment interventions, leading both to prolonged pain reporting and increased likelihood of seeking additional treatment. A recent study by McCreary et al. (1992) demonstrated that high somatization was predictive of poorer response to multidisciplinary treatment for TMD patients.

Somatization and Explanatory Models

High treatment utilization and poor response to treatment potentially arise because individuals who are highly somatically oriented hold a more biologic or physical explanatory model for their condition. As such, these patients may be less amenable to broad-based treatment approaches that emphasize the modification of specific behaviors that cause or exacerbate their pain condition.

In a preliminary study of 63 patients undergoing treatment in a TMD specialty clinic, we found an association between patients' explanatory models of TMD and scores on the SCL somatization scale. We assessed patients' global beliefs about the relative importance of physical factors, pathogenic behaviors (e.g., teeth clenching and grinding) and stress in the exacerbation and treatment of TMD symptoms. Somatization scores (with pain items removed) were positively correlated with global beliefs about the importance of physical factors in TMD ($r = 0.27$) and negatively correlated with global beliefs about the importance of pathogenic behaviors in TMD ($r = -0.33$). The observation that SCL somatization scores were higher in patients reporting primarily physical explanations of TMD and lower in patients reporting behavioral explanations of

TMD is potentially explained by the view that physical symptoms may be a somatic "idiom of expression" that focuses the report of personal and social distress on physical rather than psychological symptoms (Kleinman & Kleinman, 1985; Katon, Kleinman, & Rosen, 1981). Alternately, the tendency to explain TMD as a physically-mediated disorder may be a characteristic explanatory style (negative affectivity and/or somatosensory amplification) of the individual that reveals a predisposition to label bodily sensations as negative physical symptoms.

The review of empirical data just concluded concerning the relationship between chronic pain and somatization suggests that chronic pain conditions afford opportunities for certain individuals to focus on physical disturbances at the expense of attending to coexisting psychologic disturbance. Simultaneously, this somatic predisposition has the potential for the initiation and maintenance of treatment-seeking behaviors to alleviate those physical symptoms. As the number of somatic complaints increase, whether those somatic complaints are manifest as more than one chronic pain condition or whether they manifest as nonspecific physical symptoms other than pain, the relationship to coexisting depressive symptomatology increases, as does the amount of pain-related disability and treatment seeking. Although there is not yet sufficient empirical evidence to declare somatization a risk factor for chronic pain, the available evidence is at least consistent with this possibility for a significant minority of chronic pain patients—especially, we believe, those who evidence heightened somatization even though they do not qualify for the formal diagnosis of Somatization Disorder by present DSM-III-R criteria.

Clinical Implications: Assessment and Management Approaches

When an individual seeks medical care, the provider's primary objective is to diagnose the problem and render appropriate treatment so that the patient is protected from significant or progressive disease. Patients seeking relief from chronic pain often present with symptoms that are difficult to diagnose, including those that are vague and diffuse, as well as presenting symptoms that appear disproportionate to the degree of measurable organic pathology. These challenging diagnostic dilemmas are often further complicated by the social and emotional sequelae of chronic pain, represented as a complex web of personal and interpersonal variables (e.g., depression, social isolation, etc.) that, over time, are intricately woven into the patient's pain experience. Thus, a major challenge to the clinician working with pain patients is to assess the extent to which somatization and other psychosocial factors may coexist with and interact with the pain condition.

Because chronic pain presents as the dynamic resolution of physical, behavioral, and psychosocial influences, the management of chronic pain has expanded beyond the biomedical model to incorporate treatment strategies consistent with the current biopsychosocial understanding of chronic pain. The biomedical treatment model is primarily directed toward the goal of curing pathologic physical processes, many of which are typically obscure and resistant to measurement. By contrast, cognitive behavioral therapies, representative of the biopsychosocial treatment model, propose to modify behavior by facilitating the return to adaptive levels of activity and social function (Fordyce, Roberts, & Sternbach, 1985), as well as modify patient beliefs, attitudes, and expectancies about pain (Turk, Meichenbaum, & Genest, 1983). Thus, cognitive behavioral therapies are directed toward helping pain patients manage and cope with chronic pain such that they can learn to live productive lives despite their pain. Patients (and many of their clinicians), however, often expect that only the identification of some pathologic physical process will allow for successful treatment, resulting in complete pain remittance. To the extent that highly somatizing patients endorse explanatory models of pain that are primarily biological in orientation, these individuals, throughout their quest for that "magic bullet" or "magical biomedical cure," are at greater risk for iatrogenic disorders resulting from multiple, extensive, and invasive diagnostic and therapeutic procedures, albeit well-intended, as well as from heavy use of potentially addictive and debilitating narcotic and sedative medications.

Assessment of Somatization

Somatization often goes undetected by primary care physicians (Bridges & Goldberg, 1985). Measures for assessing somatization include the Somatosensory Amplification Scale (Barsky, Goodson,

TABLE 2.1 Explanatory Model Interview (modified) (Kleinman, 1980)

1. Beliefs About Etiology:
    What is the nature of your health problem?
    What do you call (i.e. name) your problem?
    What do you think has caused your problem?
2. Beliefs About Time and Mode of Onset:
    When did your health problem begin?
    Why do you think it started when it did?
3. Beliefs About Pathophysiology:
    How does your health problem affect your body?
    What does your illness do to your body and how does it do this?
4. Beliefs About Course of Illness:
    How severe is your health problem?
    What type of course (e.g. short or long) will it follow?
5. Treatment Expectations:
    What kind of treatment do you think you should receive for this health problem?
    What are the most important results you hope to receive from the treatment?
6. Meaning of the Symptoms:
    What do you fear most about your health problem?
    What are the chief problems your illness has caused for you?
    Why are you seeking help for this health problem now?
    How does your health problem relate to anything happening in your family, social, or work environment?

Lane, et al., 1988), the Illness Behavior Questionnaire (Pilowsky & Spence, 1983), the Somatization Subscale of the Symptom Checklist 90-Revised (Derogatis, 1983), and the Diagnostic Interview Schedule (Gardos & Cole, 1980). A review of these measures is beyond the scope of this chapter; however, a comprehensive review of many of these measures is found in a chapter on the measurement of illness behavior by Dworkin and Wilson (1992).

In clinical settings, a thorough interview aimed at understanding the patient's explanatory model, and inquiring about relevant psychiatric disorders is likely to be as useful as any currently available formal assessment. Kleinman (1980), through his efforts toward enhancing clinicians' understanding of their patient's experience of illness, has introduced a semistructured interview format for assessing explanatory models of illness (Table 2.1). Explanatory models serve as organizers of health care behaviors that influence whether an individual seeks health care services, what types of services are desired, and where and from whom the patient seeks help for relief from their symptoms. The explanatory model interview helps delineate the individual's beliefs and expectations about a specific pain episode—what causes the pain, what should be done for it, and what the pain means for overall well-being. The clinician can, therefore, gain a general understanding of whether the patient has a primarily biological explanation for his or her pain versus a psychosocial, behavioral, or mixed (e.g., a biopsychosocial model) explanatory model. This understanding will allow the clinician to (1) frame medical explanations and prescriptives to patients in terms that are consistent with the patient's explanatory model, and (2) identify discrepancies between the patient's and provider's explanatory models and search for the commonalities between these models so that various treatment strategies can be negotiated between patient and provider.

Katon (1985) has suggested that patients suspected to be somatizing should be screened for panic disorder and major depression due to the high prevalence of these conditions (7–13% and 6–10%, respectively) in primary care settings. Primary care studies have documented that 87% of the patients with psychiatric problems in primary care experience depression or anxiety. In addition, Goldberg (1979) has found that 50% of the patients with depression and anxiety present with a somatic complaint. Patients demonstrating symptoms of depression and/or anxiety are often high utilizers of health care services. Guidelines for screening for somatization among chronically ill patients are described by Katon (1985) and are summarized in Table 2.2.

Management of Somatization

Strategies for managing somatization fall into two general domains. The first domain involves elicitation, evaluation, and modification of the patient's explanatory model. The second domain aims to decrease provider behaviors which encourage somatic preoccupation and promote the "patient role."

Primary objectives in the management of somatizing patients include ensuring patient safety by preventing significant and/or progressive disease, as well as unnecessary diagnostic, invasive, or pharmacologic medical interventions. For the somatizing patient,

TABLE 2.2 Increased Risk for Somatization: Historical Factors
(Katon, 1985; Smith, Monson, & Ray, 1985)

1. Developmental histories of gross neglect, child abuse. and sexual abuse;
2. Unstable adult relationships characterized by multiple divorces and often physical violence;
3. Past family histories of alcoholism;
4. A past history of alcohol abuse prior to the start of somatization;
5. Past history of substance abuse;
6. A positive review of systems on medical history:
7. A polysurgical history;
8. A history of litigious relationships with authority figures;
9. Past history of psychiatric illness;
10. Modelling of pain behavior in their families as ways or solving problems and coping with intimate relationships.

one important vehicle for achieving these objectives is the doctor–patient relationship. A comprehensive understanding of both the patient's and the provider's explanatory model of illness is essential to the doctor–patient relationship (Kleinman, 1988). When patients' illness explanations are discrepant with their doctors', patients are likely to experience frustration with the health care system and increased anxiety about their illness (Kleinman, 1988; Turk, 1990).

Frustration with the health care system may drive patients to seek services from other clinicians who share the somatizer's primarily biologic view of their disorder. Health care providers who do not recognize their patients' somatic preoccupation and selectively attend to physical symptoms at the expense of accompanying psychological distress can unknowingly foster symptom reporting and illness behavior. Excessive symptom reporting and other illness behaviors increase patients' risk for unnecessary diagnostic procedures including potentially debilitating medical and pharmacologic interventions.

When patients are given illness explanations that they cannot effectively integrate into their existing illness model, the resulting ambiguity may increase anxiety about symptoms resulting in increased vigilance to symptoms and subsequent symptom amplification (Barsky, Geringer, & Wool, 1988). Clinicians can unwittingly inflate patients' anxiety over and vigilance to symptoms by continuing to "evaluate" and "treat" the somatizer's often vague and diffuse symptoms. Multiple diagnostic procedures with "inconclusive" test results can intensify the somatically oriented patient's anxiety about lack of detection of the correct cause of their problem, furthering their perception that opportunities for effective treatment are still beyond reach.

Conversely, difficulties in the doctor–patient relationship may also arise when clinicians focus too exclusively on the patient's psychologic distress or psychiatric status. Clinicians who subscribe to the "masked" psychiatric illness perspective, in which somatization is viewed as a psychologic defense for underlying psychologic or psychiatric disturbance, are too often viewed by their patients as unsympathetic to their illness complaints. Consequently, these patients often feel frustrated and misunderstood by their clinicians (Simon, 1991). As the doctor–patient relationship becomes strained, the clinician may, in turn, label the patient as "defensive" or "resistant," further exacerbating an already tenuous relationship. In addition, once patients are viewed as defensive or resistant by their clinicians, their somatic complaints may rate only minimal attention, and, in the worst scenario, legitimate medical care, paradoxically, may be inappropriately withheld. It is important to remember that patients who are viewed as somatizing are still at the same risk as others for becoming seriously ill.

The nonspecific amplification model of somatization does not treat physical distress as a "defense" against the real problem but as part of the real problem (Simon, 1991). In addition, within this model somatization is considered a perceptual style that is amenable to modification through cognitive and behavioral interventions. Cognitive behavioral interventions for somatic preoccupation aim to decrease the patient's vigilance toward somatic symptomatology by: (1) decreasing worry and anxiety about symptoms using patient education and provision of an alternate explanatory model, (2) effecting a shift in the patient's illness attributions and symptom-labeling process, and (3) modifying behavior by facilitating the return to adaptive levels of activity and social function (Barsky, Geringer, & Wool, 1988; Kleinman, 1988; Fordyce, Roberts, & Sternbach, 1985; Turk, Meichenbaum, & Genest, 1983). In addition, cognitive behavioral interventions usually necessitate patient involvement in design of the treatment program, thereby leading to the establishment of a collaborative relationship between clinician and patient.

Certain provider behaviors, such as inappropriate prescribing of narcotics and other medications, and directives for excessive bed rest or excessive activity limitation, have been viewed as risk factors for pain chronicity and pain-related disability. We speculate that highly somatic patients, who are often viewed as "frustrating" by their providers, may elicit these treatment directives from their providers.

There are additional provider behaviors which may also intensify patient's somatic preoccupation. As discussed earlier, provider behaviors (e.g., multiple diagnostic and treatment procedures) that focus exclusive attention on the physical or biologic aspects of vague and diffuse symptoms can (1) place patients at increased risk for potentially debilitating medical and pharmacologic interventions, and (2) increase patient anxiety about and vigilance to symptoms, particularly when diagnostic tests repeatedly demonstrate "inconclusive" results, or when multiple treatment procedures fail to eliminate the patient's symptoms.

Providers can potentially reduce patients' somatic preoccupation by minimizing the rewards associated with the "patient role" (Smith, Monson, & Ray, 1985; Simon, 1991). A salient example of this strategy is the scheduling of regularly timed appointments that are not contingent on either the occurrence of new symptoms or the worsening of old symptoms. In addition, providers can emphasize treatment based on relief of symptoms rather than repeated diagnostic exploration as a means to reduce patients' incentives to present more symptoms to receive more diagnostic tests. It is recommended that somatizing patients be assigned one provider who serves as a case manager as a way of limiting the number of providers and the potential for conflicting therapies.

Finally, providers can reduce somatization by emphasizing treatment strategies that involve patients as active participants in their health care. In particular, providers can promote treatment strategies that incorporate self-guided homework assignments, educational self-help materials (e.g., books and tapes), and community support resources as a means for decreasing patient's dependence upon the health-care system. Such strategies both enhance patients' sense of personal control over and mastery of their symptoms and convey to the patient that the provider is actively involved in symptom management and is not dismissing the patient's concerns.

It is important to keep in mind that the health care provider's behavior as a risk factor for chronic pain—especially dysfunctional chronic pain—remains largely theoretical and speculative. The notion gathers its legitimacy from clinical consensus and conventional wisdom. The health care provider's actions may undesirably influence the course of illness as well as carrying the desired promise of successful restoration of health and function. While the notion elicits an appropriate cautionary note, it must be recognized that objective data is not yet available to confirm which behaviors of health care providers are risk factors for dysfunctional chronic pain.

Summary and Conclusion

The presence of physical symptoms unexplained or inconsistent with objective physical findings tends to be interpreted by health care providers as reflecting *somatization*. Somatization Disorder, as defined by DSM-III-R provides a psychiatric diagnosis for individuals with truly abundant physical symptoms—13 or more symptoms dispersed over numerous organ systems. In fact, Somatization Disorder is a relatively rare occurrence. Of more immediate concern to primary and nonpsychiatric health-care providers is the presentation of three or more physical symptoms, also unaccompanied by pathophysiologic changes and frequently accompanied by symptoms of anxiety and/or depression.

Since pain is the most ubiquitous physical symptom, it should not be surprising that many presentations of nonspecific physical symptoms include the presentation of pain. The most important reason for considering the relationship between pain complaint and somatization relates to the possibility that when chronic pain complaints increase in number, nonspecific factors in the person may require more attention than the physical condition. Thus, the presence of numerous physical complaints, including pain, may be telling us more about the emotional and mental state of the person than about physical status.

Somatization, unlike almost all other DSM-III-R diagnostic categories, continues to require diagnosis by *interpretation* of presenting symptoms, rather than representing a diagnosis based on *description* of symptoms. The interpretation implied by the concept of somatization is that nonspecific pains and other physical symptoms represent underlying psychologic distress. Some take a psychodynamic perspective in viewing somatization as masked depression or otherwise representing a conversion of emotional upset into physical symptomatology. More recently, the cognitive behavioral perspective implies that these nonspecific physical symptoms indicate the presence of nonspecific psychological upset, reflecting widely prevalent, indeed commonly manifested, symptoms of anxiety and depression. Indeed, the view is emerging that the dichotomy between physical symptoms and psychological symptoms associated with the most common mental disorders (anxiety and depression) is an artificial one; the observed co-occurrence of abundant physical symptoms and emotional distress makes such a view appealing. Currently, there is support for the notion that certain individuals may either be predisposed to or acquire a generalized tendency to experience life events as having negative meanings and negative consequences—the term *negative affectivity* (Watson & Clark, 1984) has been introduced in this context and linked to such historically important concepts as neurasthenia and neuroticism.

In any event, it is important to remember that not all chronic pain patients could be described as somatizers, either by the stringent DSM-III-R criteria or by less stringent criteria suggested by others. However, somatization in combination with chronic pain complaints does seem to be related to the presence of increased disability and heightened patterns of treatment seeking. The possibility of somatization warrants attention from all health care providers who may be expected (by the patient) to discover, or at least evaluate, a physical condition and fix a "broken part." In fact, the patient would be at least equally well served to have attention directed to coexisting emotional distress in order to ameliorate physical and psychological symptoms, *both* of which are having a significant impact on the cognitive, emotional, and behavioral status of the patient.

References

American Dental Association, (1983). *The president's conference on the examination, diagnosis and management of temporomandibular disorders.* Chicago: American Dental Association.
American Psychiatric Association, (1987). *Diagnostic and statistical manual*

of mental disorders. (3rd edition, revised). Washington, DC: American Psychiatric Association Press.

Barsky, A. J. (1979). Patients who amplify bodily sensations. *Annals of Internal Medicine, 91*, 63–70.

Barsky, A. J., Geringer, E., & Wool, C. A. (1988). A cognitive educational treatment for hypochondriasis. *General Hospital Psychiatry, 10*, 1–6.

Barsky, A. J., Goodson, J. D., Lane, R. S., et al, (1988). The amplification of somatic symptoms. *Psychosomatic Medicine, 50*, 510–519.

Blumer, D., & Heilbronn, M. (1982). Chronic pain as a variant of depressive disease. *Journal of Nervous and Mental Disease, 170*, 381–406.

Bridges, K. W., & Goldberg, D. P. (1985). Somatic presentation of DSM III psychiatric disorders in primary care. *Journal of Psychosomatic Research, 29*, 563–569.

Chrisman, N. (1977). The health seeking process: An approach to the natural history of illness. *Culture Medicine and Psychiatry, 1*, 351–377.

Derogatis, L. R. (1983). *SCL-90-R: Administration, scoring and procedures manual—II for the revised version*. Towson, MD: Clinical Psychometric Research.

Dworkin, S. F., LeResche, L., & Von Korff, M. (1989). Studying the natural history of TMD: Epidemiologic perspectives on physical and psychological findings. In K. D. Vig & P. S. Vig (Eds.). *Clinical research as the basis for clinical practice* (pp. 39–60). Ann Arbor, MI: University of Michigan.

Dworkin, S. F., Von Korff, M., & LeResche, L. (1990). Multiple pains and psychiatric disturbance: An epidemiologic investigation. *Archives of General Psychiatry, 47*, 239–244.

Dworkin, S. F., Von Korff, M. R., & LeResche, L. (1992). Epidemiologic studies of chronic pain: A dynamic-ecologic perspective. *Annals of Behavioral Medicine, 14*, 3–11.

Dworkin, S. F., & Wilson, L. (1992). Measurement of illness behavior: Review of concepts and common measures. In *Methods in neurosciences*. San Diego (in press): Academic.

Eisenberg, L. (1986). Mindlessness and brainlessness in psychiatry. *British Journal of Psychiatry, 148*, 457–508.

Escobar, J. I., Jacqueline, M. G., Hough, R. L., Karno, M., Burnam, M. A., & Wells, K. B. (1987). Somatization in the community: Relationship to disability and use of services. *American Journal of Public Health, 77*(7), 837–840.

Escobar, J. I., Burnam, A., Karno, M., Forsythe, A., & Golding, J. M. (1987). Somatization in the community. *Archives of General Psychiatry, 44*, 713–718.

Fletcher, R. H., Fletcher, S. W. & Wagner, E. H. (1988). *Clinical epidemiology: The essentials*. Baltimore: Williams & Wilkins.

Fordyce, W. E. (1976). *Behavioral methods in chronic pain and illness*. St. Louis, MO: Mosby.

Fordyce, W. E., Roberts, A. H., & Sternbach, R. A. (1985). The behavioral management of chronic pain: A response to critics. *Pain, 22,* 113–125.

Gardos, G., & Cole, J. O. (1980). Problems in the assessment of tardive dyskinesia. In W. E. Fann, R. C. Smith, J. M. Davis, & E. F. Domino (Eds.). *Tardive Dyskinesia: Research and treatment* (pp. 201–214). New York: Domino.

Gil, K. M., Phillips, G., Abrams, M. R., & Williams, D. A. (1990). Pain drawings and sickle cell disease pain. *Clinical Journal of Pain, 6,* 105–109.

Goldberg, D. (1979). Detection and assessment of emotional disorders in a primary care setting. *International Journal of Mental Health, 8,* 30–48.

Goldberg, D., & Huxley, P. (1992). *Common mental disorders: A bio-social model.* London: Tavistock/Routledge.

Greene, C. L., & Marbach, J. J. (1982). Epidemiologic studies of mandibular dysfunction: A critical view. *Journal of Prosthetic Dentistry, 48,* 184–190.

Katon, W. (1985). Somatization in primary care. *Journal of Family Practice, 21*(4), 257–258.

Katon, W., Lin, E., Von Korff, M., Russo, J., Lipscomb, P., & Bush, T. (1991). Somatization: A spectrum of severity. *American Journal of Psychiatry, 148,* 34–40.

Katon, W., Kleinman, A., & Rosen, G. (1981). Depression and somatization: A review, part II. *American Journal of Medicine, 72,* 241–247.

Ketterer, M. W., & Buckholtz, C. D. (1989). Somatization disorder. *Journal of the American Osteopathic Association, 89,* 489–499.

Kleinman, A. (1980). *Patients and healers in the context of culture: An exploration of the borderland between anthropology, medicine and psychiatry.* Berkeley: University of California Press.

Kleinman, A. (1988). *The illness narratives: Suffering, healing and the human condition.* New York: Basic Books.

Kleinman, A., & Kleinman, J. (1985). Somatization: Interconnections between Chinese culture, depressive meanings and the experience of pain. In A. Kleinman & B. Good (Eds.). *Culture and depression.* Berkeley: University of California Press.

Litman, T. J. (1974). The family as a basic unit in health and medical care. *Social Science and Medicine, 8,* 495–519.

Loeser, J. D. (1980). Perspectives on pain. In *Proceedings of the First World Congress on Clinical Pharmacology and Therapeutics* (pp. 313–316). London: Macmillan.

McCreary, C. P., Clark, G. T., Oakley, M. E., & Flack, V. (1992). Predicting response to treatment for Temporomandibular Disorders. *Journal of Craniomandibular Disorders: Facial & Oral Pain, 6,* 161–170.

Mechanic, D. (1986). Illness behavior: An overview. In S. McHugh & T. M. Vallis (Eds.). *Illness behavior: A multidisciplinary model.* New York: Plenum.

Melzack, R., & Wall, P. D. (1965). Pain mechanisms: A new theory. *Science, 150,* 971–979.

Moss, R. A., Garrett, J., & Chiodo, J. F. (1982). Temporomandibular joint dysfunction and myofascial pain dysfunction syndromes: Parameters, etiology, and treatment. *Psychological Bulletin, 92*, 331–346.

Parsons, T. (1975). The sick role and the role of the physician reconsidered. *Milbank Memorial Fund Quarterly, 53*, 257–278.

Pilowsky, I., Spence, N., Cobb, J., & Katsikitis, M. (1984). The illness behavior questionnaire as an aid to clinical assessment. *General Hospital Psychiatry, 6*, 123–130.

Pilowsky, I., & Spence, N. D. (1983). *Manual for the Illness Behaviour Questionnaire (IBQ)*. Adelaide: University of Adelaide.

Romano, J. M., & Turner, J. A. (1985). Chronic pain and depression: Does the evidence support a relationship? *Psychological Bulletin, 97*, 18–26.

Rudy, T. E., Turk, D. C., Zaki, H. S., & Curtin, H. D. (1989). An empirical taxometric alternative to traditional classification of temporomandibular disorders. *Pain, 36*, 311–320.

Schwartz, D. P., & DeGood, D. E. (1984). Global appropriateness of pain drawings: Blind ratings predict patterns of psychological distress and litigation status. *Pain, 19*, 383–388.

Simon, G. E. (1991). Somatization and psychiatric disorders. In L. J. Kirmayer & J. M. Bobbins (Eds.), *Current concepts of somatization: Research and clinical perspectives* (31st ed.) (pp. 37–62). Washington, DC: American Psychiatric Press.

Smith, G., Monson, R. A., & Ray, D. C. (1985). Psychiatry consultation in somatization disorder: A randomized controlled study. *Presented at Forty-second Annual Meeting of the American Psychosomatic Society Washington, DC.*

Smith, G. R., Munson, R. A., & Ray, D. C. (1986). Patients with multiple unexplained symptoms. *Archives of Internal Medicine, 146*, 69–72.

Swartz, M., Blazer, D., Woodbury, M., George, L., & Landerman, R. (1986). Somatization disorder in a US southern community: Use of a new procedure for analysis of medical classification. *Psychological Medicine, 16*, 595–609.

Toomey, T. C., Cover, V. F., & Jones, B. N. (1983). Spatial distribution of pain: A descriptive characteristic of chronic pain. *Pain, 17*, 289–300.

Turk, D., & Flor, H. (1987). Pain pain behaviors: The utility of the pain behavior construct. *Pain, 31*, 277–295.

Turk, D.C. (1990). Customizing treatment for chronic pain patients: Who, what, why. *Clinical Journal of Pain, 6*, 255–270.

Turk, D. C., Meichenbaum, D., & Genest, M. (1983). *Pain and behavioral medicine. A cognitive behavioral perspective.* New York: Guilford.

Von Korff, M., Ormel, J., Keefe, F. J., & Dworkin, S. F. (1992). Grading the severity of chronic pain. *Pain, 50*, 133–149.

Von Korff, M. R. (1992). Epidemiologic and survey methods: Chronic pain assessment. In D. C. Turk & R. Melzack (Eds.). *Handbook of pain assessment.* New York: Guilford.

Von Korff, M. R., Dworkin, S. F., LeResche, L., & Kruger, A. (1988). An epidemiologic comparison of pain complaints. *Pain, 32,* 173–183.

Watson, D., & Clark, L. A. (1984). Negative affectivity: The disposition to experience aversive emotional states. *Psychological Bulletin, 96*(3), 465–490.

Wilson, L., Dworkin, S. F., Whitney, C., & LeResche, L. (in press) Somatization and pain dispersion in chronic temporomandibular disorder pain. *Pain.*

Chapter Three

Muscle Overuse and Posture as Factors in the Development and Maintenance of Chronic Musculoskeletal Pain

Susan J. Middaugh, William G. Kee, and
John A. Nicholson

Painful musculoskeletal disorders are a major cause of lost produc-
tivity, work-related disability, and employee health care costs (Cunningham & Kelsey, 1984; Frymoyer & Cats-Baril, 1991; Sternbach,
1986). In 1983, for example, 24% of sick-leave days in Sweden were
due to pain in the back, neck, and shoulders (Kellett, Kellett, &
Nordholm, 1991). At present, there is considerable interest in muscle overuse as a major factor in the development and maintenance
of work-related musculoskeletal pain. This interest is due to high,
and rapidly increasing, rates of musculoskeletal pain problems in
categories of workers that were not previously considered to be at
risk including office workers and workers performing relatively
light manufacturing tasks such as assembly of electronic components. In these workers, job-related injuries are usually not due to a
single acute event such as a fall or lifting a heavy object. Rather,
the problem is one of cumulative trauma arising from long-term
overload of muscles and other soft tissues (tendons, ligaments,
nerve sheaths) due to factors such as work posture, speed, and repetitiveness. In the relevant clinical and research literature, these
musculoskeletal pain disorders are commonly termed cumulative

trauma disorder (CTD), repetitive strain injury (RSI) or overuse syndrome (OS).

In recent years, overuse injury has become the fastest growing category of workplace injury. According to the Bureau of Labor statistics, such injuries accounted for nearly half of all workplace illnesses in private industry in 1988, compared to only 18% in 1981 (Kantrowitz & Crandall, 1990). The Occupational Safety and Health Administration (OSHA) has observed a 100% increase in CTD claims each year in recent years. At present, this problem strikes an estimated 185,000 workers a year and costs an estimated $7 billion annually in lost productivity and medical costs (Hebert, 1990; Horowitz, 1992). Overuse syndromes are now recognized by the medical community as a serious, and growing, medical problem (Kasden, 1991; Millender, Louis, & Simmons, 1992; Putz-Anderson, 1988; Soderberg, 1992).

It is interesting that the current increase has largely come from office workers, particularly those whose jobs require extensive keyboard operation at video display terminals (VDTs) for word processing, data entry, and other computer-automated tasks (Hagberg & Wegman, 1987; Kantrowitz, 1990).

There is a large pool of workers whose jobs include VDT operation due to an accelerating trend toward office automation and information processing, and there are a number of characteristics of VDT operation that place these workers at risk of overuse injuries (Arndt, 1983): (1) VDT operators spend lengthy periods of time in postures that place a static load on the muscles, particularly in the cervical and shoulder girdle area, producing rapid muscle fatigue (Chaffin, 1973; Onishi, Nomura, & Sakai, 1973); (2) job tasks include simplified repetitive motion patterns that overuse the muscles, tendons, and joints and irritate connective tissue sheaths surrounding the nerves; (3) speed, automation, and monotony increase factors such as time pressure, emotional stress, and job dissatisfaction that in turn contribute to symptom development (Kilbom, Persson, & Johnsson, 1985; Smith, Cohen, Stammerjohn, & Happ, 1981; Smith, Stammerjohn, Cohen, & Lalich, 1980). The result is a high rate of tension-type headache, pain in the cervical, shoulder girdle, and back areas, and carpal tunnel syndrome.

To date, the predominant approach to research and intervention has been to use anthropomorphic measurements, engineering assessments, and physiological recording procedures, particularly electromyography (EMS), to determine the postures, joint loads. and required muscle forces for specific job tasks. This information is then used to redesign work stations and work tasks to make them more ergonomically correct (Corlett, Wilson, & Manenica, 1985; Kilbom et al., 1985; Soderberg, 1992). Such design changes have led to substantial reductions in musculoskeletal pain problems in a number of industrial areas (Aaras, Westgaard, & Stranden, 1988).

The problem with this approach is that it focuses almost exclusively on *work-site characteristics*. Work-station design (e.g., placement of the VDT keyboard or screen) and work task characteristics (e.g., repetitiveness and speed) are seen as imposing faulty work postures and excessive task demands on the operator. From this point of view, the solution is simply to redesign the work station and alter the task requirements and thereby prevent or remediate the overuse problem.

Relatively little research has been directed toward *operator characteristics* as important variables in the development or correction of overuse syndromes. The individual operator has a set of acquired postures, habitual patterns of muscle use, and psychosocial/ life-style characteristics that determine, in part, how that individual interacts with the work environment. Kilbom et al. (1985) found that workers who developed carpal tunnel syndrome were more likely to engage in home hobbies such as knitting that involved repetitive hand activities. Other investigators have reported correlations between CTD, job stress, and job dissatisfaction (Smith et al., 1981). We have reported (Middaugh, 1992; Middaugh & Kee, 1987) that factors such as forward head posture and habitual patterns of muscle overuse can lead to prolonged muscle contractions in cervical and shoulder girdle muscles that continue during the "rest" portion of work/rest cycles. A very interesting videographic study of electronics workers (Kilbom et al., 1985) found that individual workers showed wide variations in the postures and movements used to carry out similar tasks. Furthermore, those workers who had pain in the cervical or shoulder girdle area made fewer postural changes and spent a greater percentage of the work cycle with the neck flexed, shoulders elevated, and upper arm flexed or abducted. These work postures place an excessive work load on the muscles in the reported area of pain. Yet there are relatively few published reports of interventions specifically designed

to alter such operator characteristics, either to prevent or to remediate muscle overuse symptoms (Middaugh, 1989; Middaugh &
Kee, 1987; Middaugh, Woods, Kee, Harden, & Peters, 1991).

There is, then, a need for research which investigates *operator
characteristics* as causative and/or contributory factors in cumulative trauma disorders. In this chapter, we examine two interrelated
operator characteristics that are implicated in the development
and maintenance of musculoskeletal pain in the head, neck, and
shoulder girdle areas: (1) inappropriate patterns of muscle use, and
(2) poor posture. In addition, we present an intervention strategy
that is designed to correct these two problems through a combination of EMG biofeedback and therapeutic exercise.

Work Posture, Muscle Overuse, and Muscle Fatigue

In a recent study carried out in our lab, Barker and Sellers (1991)
investigated the impact of work posture on the upper trapezius
muscle. This is a key muscle that participates in many different
movements of the head and neck and that stabilizes the scapula
during activities involving the upper extremity (arm and hand). It
is a very common site of pain symptoms and trigger points in the
cervical and shoulder girdle area and is also thought to play a substantial role in tension-type headache (Middaugh, 1989; Middaugh
& Garwood, 1989; Travell & Simons, 1983).

Twenty normal, healthy college students with good upper body
posture participated in this study. Good posture was defined as less
than 10 degrees of forward head posture with no fixed postural abnormalities such as kyphosis. Subjects had no remarkable muscle
soreness in the trapezius muscle on manual palpation and no history of recurrent headaches, musculoskeletal problems, or injuries
to the head, neck, or shoulder girdle area.

All subjects participated in a single experimental session in
which they typed at their typical speed at a computer keyboard for 15
minutes, rested for 5 minutes, and then repeated the 15-minute typing task. During one of the 15-minute typing periods, each subject
worked in an ergonomically correct posture (Fig. 3.1) defined as sitting with zero degrees of shoulder flexion and shoulder abduction and
90 degrees elbow flexion. This placed the elbow at the side of the trunk
and the forearm parallel to the floor when the fingers were placed on

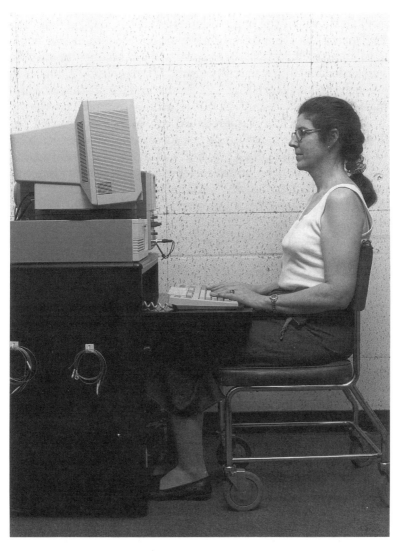

FIGURE 3.1   Ergonomically correct work posture for keyboard operation.

the keyboard. The feet were flat on the floor with hips and knees at 90 degrees of flexion, and the chair was adjusted for good lumbar trunk support. During the other 15-minute typing period, the same subject worked in an altered posture that required 30 degrees of forward flexion at the shoulder (and a corresponding 120 degrees of elbow extension) to reach the keyboard (Fig. 3.2). Trunk and leg posture remained unchanged. This is a substantial, but relatively common, postural deviation that occurs when the keyboard operator is not seated close enough to the computer terminal (as, for example, when the chair arms do not fit under the desk top) and has to reach forward to touch the keys. The order of presentation of the two typing tasks was counterbalanced to control for possible order effects.

Muscle activity was recorded electromyographically using the Advanced Technology AT33* (20–560 Hz bandwidth), which provides a single channel of EMG recording and quantification. Surface electrodes were placed over the right upper trapezius muscle at the shoulder (Fig. 3.3). EMG was quantified as mean microvolts (rms) for an initial 1-minute baseline (hands resting in the lap), for sequential 1-minute periods throughout the 15-minute typing tasks, and for a final 1-minute baseline (hands once again in the lap).

The results are illustrated in Fig. 3.4. Mean EMG during the first minute of typing was greater for the ALTERED work position than for the ERGONOMIC position ($p < .01$), indicating that a substantially stronger muscle contraction was required to perform the typing task in poor working posture. In addition, mean EMG increased from minute 1 to minute 15 ($p < .01$) of the typing task for the incorrect posture, indicating the development of muscle fatigue: as a muscle fatigues during a continuous, submaximal task such as the typing task in this study, mean EMG voltage increases (Basmajian & De Luca, 1985; Enoka & Stuart, 1992; Hagberg & Kvarnstrom, 1984; Soderberg, 1992). There was no such indication of muscle fatigue when typing was performed in the ergonomically correct posture.

This relatively simple study in a nonpatient population illustrates clearly that poor working posture, in this case due to incorrect placement of the keyboard, can result in significant muscle overuse. That is, the muscle contraction required to perform the work task with poor working posture far exceeded the muscle contraction required to perform the same task when carried out with the ergonomically correct work posture. Furthermore, this muscle overuse led to the rapid development of localized muscle fatigue.

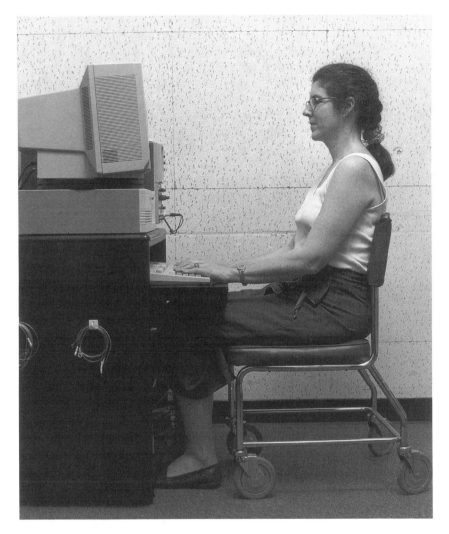

FIGURE 3.2 Altered work posture for keyboard operation, with 30 degrees of shoulder forward flexion.

Habitual Posture and Muscle Overuse in Headache and Cervical-Pain Patients

The problematic work posture in the preceding study was induced by the short-term demands of a specific work station arrangement

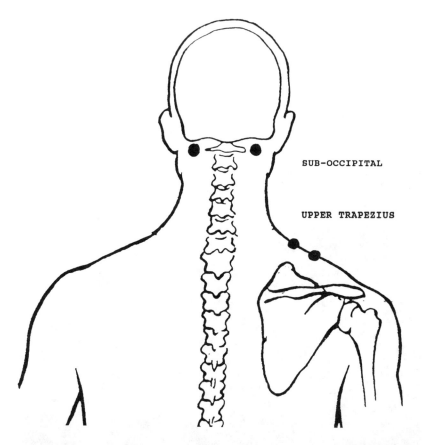

FIGURE 3.3 Electrode placements for surface EMG recording at two sites, the Upper Trapezius muscle and the sub-occipital muscles.

and was easily corrected by changing the position of the keyboard. There is, however, a second source of incorrect work posture that is considerably more difficult to identify and reverse; namely, the individual worker's habitual body posture. Habitual posture is relatively stable, is present across many different tasks, has a profound effect on muscle use, and is relatively difficult to change, particularly since muscles adapt by becoming shortened (and tight) or lengthened (and weak) to fit habitual joint positions.

Figs. 3.5 and 3.6 illustrate a problem with habitual head posture that we find to be very common in patients with chronic tension-type

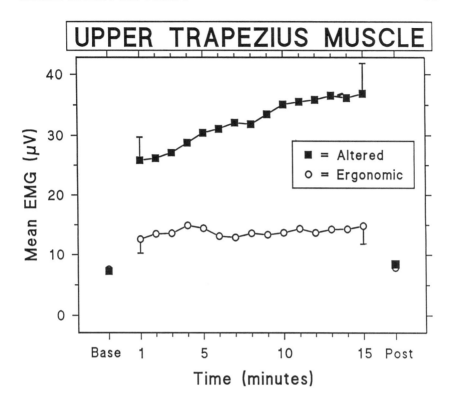

FIGURE 3.4 EMG recorded over the Upper Trapezius ms of a single group of 20 subjects during 15 minutes of continuous keyboard operation in two different work postures; an ergonomically correct posture and an altered posture with 30 degrees of forward shoulder flexion.

headache: *forward head posture*, in which the head is displaced forward of the body's center of gravity in the sagittal plane. This head position can be measured as the angle between an imaginary plumb line running through the acromion process of the shoulder, and a second line running between the acromion and the auditory meatus of the ear. There is good agreement in textbooks on human anatomy and kinesiology that the ideal is zero degrees of forward head position, with the ear centered directly above the shoulder (Fig. 3.5). There is less information on what constitutes an acceptable deviation from this ideal. The infor-

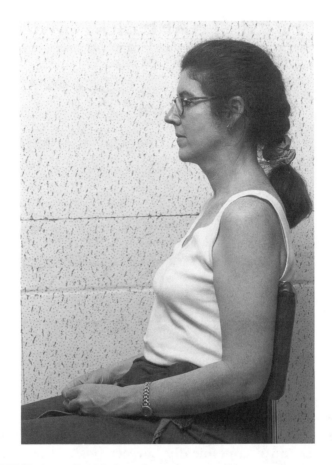

FIGURE 3.5 Good head posture: the ear is centered above the shoulder with the auditory meatus 0–5 degrees forward of the acromion process of the shoulder.

mation provided with the Scan-A-Graph (TM)*, a device for quantitative measurement of posture in clinical settings, states that 7 degrees of forward head posture is the start of moderate deviation and 12 degrees is the start of marked deviation, but the source of these values is not referenced. Textbook illustrations of individuals with marked forward head posture (as in Fig. 3.6) are usually approximately 15 degrees.

*TM: Postural Scan-A-Graph, Reedco Research, 51 N., Auburn N.Y., 13021.

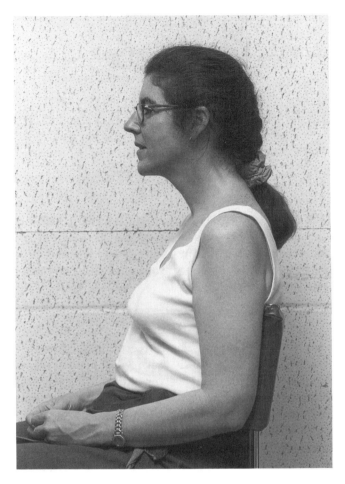

FIGURE 3.6 A forward head posture of 15 degrees: The auditory meatus of the ear is 15 degrees forward of the acromion process of the shoulder.

The relevance of forward head posture for patients with cervical pain and headache is illustrated in Figure 3.7. This is a polygraph tracing of raw EMG recorded from electrodes placed over the right and left suboccipital muscle group at the base of the skull. These muscles act (with other neck muscles) to position and move the head on the cervical spine. The upper trapezius muscle overlies the deeper suboccipital muscles but it consists almost entirely of connective tissue near the base of

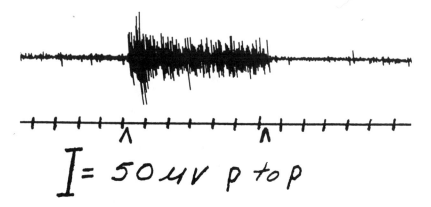

I = 50 μV p to p

FIGURE 3.7 Raw EMG recording from the sub-occipital ms site: the subject sits with good head posture (left), then assumes and holds a 15 degree forward head posture for 6 seconds (between markers), then resumes good head posture (right).

the skull and does not contribute to the surface recorded EMG with appropriate electrode placement. The EMG tracing begins at left, with a normal individual sitting quietly with good head posture (approximately 5 degrees). EMG activity is very low but increases strongly as the subject assumes a pronounced forward head posture (approximately 15 degrees). At right, the EMG decreases back to a low level when the subject resumes the initial good head posture. One can see the substantial workload that forward head posture places on the muscles of the posterior cervical area at the base of the skull. Habitual forward head posture, therefore, can produce marked overuse of these muscles, which are a common site of reported pain in many patients with chronic tension-type headache and cervical pain.

Table 3.1 presents data from 35 consecutive headache patients (7 male, 28 female, Mean age = 40 years, range = 19–79 years) evaluated at the Medical University of South Carolina (MUSC) Chronic Pain Rehabilitation Program (CPRP). Patients were diagnosed by a neurologist as having chronic tension-type or mixed headache ($N = 26$, 74.3%), vascular headache ($N = 4$, 11.4%), or other headache diagnoses ($N = 5$, 14%). Cervical active range of motion (AROM) and forward head position were measured by a physical therapist using an arthrodial protractor for rotation and a goniometer for forward head position and lateral flex-

TABLE 3.1   Cervical Active Range of Motion and Head Posture in
Headache Patients (N = 35)

Degrees of AROM:	Rotation	Lateral Flex	Forward Head Posture
Headache Patients	53°	28°	16°
Cervical Orthopedic	52°	27°	
Normative Data	65°–80°	35°–45°	7°–10°
Percent Deviation in Headache Pts.	18%–34%	20%–38%	128%–60%

ion. Also in Table 3.1 are comparable data reported in the literature:
the mean AROM reported for a group of orthopedic patients seeking
treatment for cervical pain (Youdas, Carey, & Garrett, 1991) and the
range of mean AROM values reported in normative studies of nonpatient groups (Alund & Larsson, 1990; Raab, Agre, McAdam, & Smith,
1988; Youdas, Garrett, Suman, Bodard, Hallman, & Carey, 1992). The
headache patients averaged 53 degrees of cervical rotation and 28 degrees of lateral cervical flexion, which is almost identical to the reported values for cervical orthopedic patients and which represents an
18% to 34% loss of active range of motion compared with published,
nonpatient norms. In addition, the headache patients averaged 16 degrees of forward head posture, which is 60% to 128% greater than values considered to be clinically significant deviations (7°–10°). Forward
head posture in the headache group ranged from 4 degrees to 25 degrees, with only 9% measured at 0–10 degrees; 44% measured at 11–15
degrees; and 47% measured at 16 degrees or greater.

These findings provide evidence of substantial problems with
habitual forward head posture and tight cervical muscles (decreased AROM) in persons with chronic headache. Both of these
problems strongly suggest that there is chronic overuse of cervical
muscles in these headache patients as well.

Static and Dynamic Patterns of Muscle Use in Headache and Cervical Pain Patients

EMG data from three separate studies (Middaugh, 1992; Middaugh
& Gee, 1987) are summarized in Table 3.2. In each of these studies,
EMG electrodes were placed over the surface of the upper trapezius

TABLE 3.2 Frequency of Electromyographic Findings

	Normal N = 32	Cervical N = 20	Headache N = 35
Elevated Sitting Baseline	25%	65%	57%
Delayed Relaxation After:			
Shoulder Shrug	9%	85%	94%
Shoulder Abduction	19%	90%	86%
Poor Relaxation on Request			
(sitting)	0%	-	50%
Elevated Standing Baseline	34%	-	83%
Poor Relaxation on Request			
(Standing)	9%	-	69%

muscle, which is a common site of musculoskeletal pain reported by patients evaluated in our pain program with chronic cervical or shoulder girdle pain or chronic headache. This electrode placement primarily records activity of the upper trapezius muscle, but it also includes some contribution from the underlying levator scapulae muscle. Both muscles elevate the shoulder and also stabilize the scapula during forward flexion or abduction of the shoulder, arm movements that occur with many different hand activities. EMG was recorded separately for the right and left using a two-channel TECA clinical EMG with oscilloscope display and tape recorder. The raw EMG signals were tape recorded during a standard protocol developed to evaluate both static and dynamic patterns of muscle use during six test activities. The EMG signals were later replayed and quantified in terms of peak-to-peak amplitude with reference to a grid on the oscilloscope screen using operationally defined criteria (given below). The initial study was carried out with 20 consecutive patients (7 male, 13 female, mean age = 44.7 years, range = 24–75 years) with chronic cervical pain and included only the first three test movements. This study is described in more detail elsewhere (Middaugh & Kee, 1987). Subsequently, the study was repeated, with three additional test movements, on 32 healthy, pain-free individuals (16 male, 16 female, mean age = 37 yr, range = 22–67 years). Finally, a third study was carried out with 35 patients with chronic headache (described above and in Table 3.1). No statistical comparisons were made, since the data for

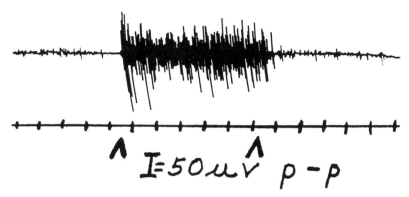

FIGURE 3.8 Normal onset and offset of voluntary muscle contraction: raw EMG (20–1000 Hz) recorded from the Upper Trapezius ms site. The subject is sitting still (left), then asked to "shrug your shoulder up and hold" (first marker), then "let go" (second marker). The muscle relaxes within 2 seconds.

the three groups were from three separate studies with some variation in procedures and sample characteristics.

As shown in Table 3.2 a high percentage of the two patient groups, but not the normal group, showed elevated EMG during quiet sitting, which indicates a degree of constant, isometric muscle contraction in the area of pain. Elevation is operationally defined as 25 microvolts or greater, peak-to-peak. An even higher percentage of the patient groups (85%–94%) showed delayed relaxation following brief, voluntary muscle contraction (3-second shoulder shrug or 3-second shoulder abduction to horizontal). Figure 3.8 illustrates a trial in which there is rapid and relatively complete muscle relaxation of the upper trapezius muscle following a brief, voluntary shoulder shrug ("shrug your shoulders up and hold; now let go"). Figure 3.9 illustrates a trial that meets the operational definition of "delayed relaxation," in which relaxation is incomplete (25 microvolts or greater, peak-to-peak) 15 seconds after the instruction "now let go." In addition to a high rate of delayed relaxation, many of the headache patients were not able to voluntarily relax the active muscle on request while sitting (50%) or while standing (69%), while few (0%–9%) normal individuals

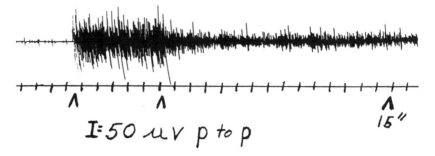

$I = 50 \mu V \ p \ to \ p$ $15''$

FIGURE 3.9 Delayed relaxation after shoulder shrug: raw EMG (20–1000 Hz) recorded from the Upper Trapezius ms site. Instructions are the same as Fig. 3.8. After instructions to "let go" (second marker), the muscle continues to contract, 25 microvolts or greater, for 15 seconds or longer.

had problems with this task. Poor relaxation on request is defined as an EMG value of 25 microvolts or more, 15 seconds after the instructions, "now think about your shoulders and let them relax." These data indicate that patients with chronic cervical/shoulder girdle pain or chronic tension type/mixed headache have a substantial problem with overuse and poor voluntary control of key muscles in the cervical area.

EMG Biofeedback Interventions to Correct Muscle Overuse

The studies presented above indicate that individuals with chronic headache or pain in the cervical area have a high incidence of three problems: muscle overuse, forward head posture, and tight cervical muscles (decreased AROM). These three problems tend to interact and reinforce each other. Poor posture can lead to overuse of some muscle groups (and underuse of their antagonists). Muscles that are used excessively become shortened and tight, as in the familiar example of tight leg muscles in distance runners. A shortened, tight muscle can in turn be difficult to relax if the relaxed position places the muscle on a stretch and, via stretch reflexes, provokes protective contraction. Also, tight muscles (in combination with their underused, weakened antagonists) can make it difficult to assume and maintain correct posture. Therefore, a successful treatment approach needs to address all three of these interrelated problems.

The treatment program at MUSC emphasizes use of EMG biofeedback procedures to reduce muscle overuse and to teach correct posture. The biofeedback procedures are combined with a therapeutic exercise program designed to stretch the tight, overused muscles and to strengthen the weakened, underused muscles to restore normal AROM and use of these muscles for posture and daily activities.

EMG biofeedback training can be very effective in correcting overuse of the upper trapezius muscles in patients with headache and cervical pain. During EMG biofeedback training, EMG signals from the target muscle or muscle group are recorded, amplified, and converted into an auditory or visual signal that varies in proportion to the voltage generated by the contracting muscle. The patient can, in effect, see or hear the muscle contract and can use the feedback signal to guide trial and error efforts to learn improved muscle control. The training begins with learning to relax the upper trapezius muscle during quiet sitting and then progresses to learning to relax the muscles quickly and reliably during repeated contract/relax cycles. The training then shifts to practice of improved muscle control during a variety of daily activities including standing, walking, simulated driving, and work-related tasks such as keyboard operation and writing. For tasks that require little use of this target muscle, the training goal is to maintain muscle relaxation during task performance. For tasks that do require use of the target muscle, the training goal is to perform the task with no greater contraction than the task actually requires and to relax the muscles rapidly to reestablish appropriate work/rest cycles. Portable biofeedback units are used for much of the training, which continues until mastery is achieved first with, and then without, the feedback signals.

The effectiveness of EMG biofeedback training is illustrated by EMG data from 14 patients with chronic cervical pain (aged 29–78 years, 8 female, 6 male) included in a recently published study (Middaugh et al., 1991). EMG evaluation (as in Table 3.2) was carried out before, and repeated after, treatment that included extensive EMG biofeedback training of the upper trapezius muscles as described above. Prior to training, 11 (79%) of the patients showed elevated sitting baseline and/or delayed relaxation after shoulder shrug. Following biofeedback training, only 2 (14%) had either of these signs of muscle overuse. These data indicate that EMG biofeedback training can effectively retrain muscle control in individuals with well-established patterns of muscle overuse.

EMG feedback, with electrodes placed over the suboccipital muscles (approximately 1 cm to the right and left of center at the level of C2, see Fig. 3.3) is also used to retrain correct neutral head position in individuals with forward head posture. The patient learns the correct balanced head position guided by the EMG feedback signal. Recorded EMG is minimal in a balanced head position and increases with forward head positions. This control is practiced while sitting, standing, and walking using portable biofeedback units. It is usually necessary to include exercises designed to systematically stretch and strengthen the cervical and shoulder girdle muscles. These exercises are carried out by the patient on a daily basis at home, and biofeedback training of the suboccipital muscles is delayed until this therapeutic exercise program is well underway.

Implications for Prevention and Treatment of Overuse Syndromes

The preceding studies point out the substantial impact on key muscle groups in the head and neck area of relatively simple positional and postural factors. A work station that is well designed and adjusted to meet the ergonomic requirements of the individual worker is necessary, but is not sufficient, to solve many problems of muscle overuse. Our studies point to at least three sources of problems that are dependent not on *work-station characteristics*, but on *operator characteristics*; that is, on the characteristics of the individual worker who performs the job.

The first source of problems is the way the worker chooses to adjust the work station. In the simplest case, the worker who reaches forward to place their fingers on a computer keyboard produces a major change in the muscle requirements of the task. This increases the work load on the cervical and shoulder girdle muscles and begins with the first inch of reach. While this problem can be caused by a work station fault such as chair arms that prevent sitting close to the desk, this problem is often simply a result of choices the worker makes in arranging their chair and keyboard within the work station. EMG biofeedback procedures can demonstrate to the worker, in a very concrete way, the physiological consequences of these choices.

A second source of problems is the habitual posture of the worker performing the task. As illustrated in Figure 3.7 above, forward head posture places an increased work load on the posterior occipital muscles. There is no work-station adjustment that will correct this problem; instead, the adjustment must be in the worker's posture. If the forward head posture has been present for a long time, it will be accompanied by tight, shortened muscles in the neck, chest, and anterior shoulder girdle areas and also weak, overstretched muscles in the posterior shoulder girdle area. The individual is usually unaware of the extent of the postural deviation which now feels "normal." Correction requires a systematic exercise program designed to stretch tight muscles and strengthen weak ones to make it possible for the worker to assume and maintain the correct posture. In addition, it is essential to train the individual to recognize and voluntarily assume the desired, balanced head position, and this can be accomplished very nicely with EMG biofeedback-assisted postural retraining.

A third source of problems lies in the habitual patterns of muscle use of the individual worker. In the studies above, there is a high incidence of habitual overuse of the upper trapezius/levator scapulae muscles in individuals with chronic cervical pain or chronic headache. This overuse is well-ingrained and out of proportion to task demands. Overuse is apparent as elevated EMG during quiet sitting and standing, two activities that normally require very little activity in these muscles. Overuse is also seen as delayed relaxation following contraction; that is, the muscle contraction persists long after the task ends. Most tasks involve sequences of contract/relax cycles, and blood flow to the muscle increases during the brief periods of relaxation to replenish energy stores. The muscle that continues to "work" during the "rest" portion of a task is at substantial risk of early fatigue. This pattern of muscle overuse can be particularly difficult to correct since many individuals are not aware of the problem and cannot readily relax these problem muscles when they initially attempt to do so. Correction requires considerable training that includes learning to relax the problem muscles during quiet sitting and standing, learning to relax the muscles rapidly during contract/relax cycles, learning to maintain muscle relaxation during tasks that do not in fact require the use of these specific muscles, and learning to contract the muscle no more than is needed during tasks that do require these muscles. As noted above, when habitual muscle overuse is accompanied by muscle tightness and corresponding underuse and weakness of antagonist muscle groups, a therapeutic exercise program is also required.

EMG monitoring and EMG feedback offers an effective method for evaluating and correcting these three sources of muscle overuse. EMG monitoring can clarify the impact on the muscles of alternative work station arrangements and thereby detect, and correct, common causes of muscle overuse. EMG monitoring can also assess patterns of muscle use, and overuse, in the individual who is having problems with musculoskeletal pain or headache. EMG biofeedback training can provide an effective method to reestablish normal contract/relax (work/rest) cycles in problem muscles and teach efficient use of overused muscles during daily activities and work-related tasks. EMG biofeedback procedures can also be used to teach the individual how to recognize and correct problem head and body postures.

The findings of the studies presented above provide ample evidence of substantial muscle overuse in patients with chronic cervical/shoulder girdle pain or chronic headache. This is accompanied, at least in the headache patients, by forward head posture. This muscle overuse and poor posture are well-ingrained and supported by a number of secondary factors, such as muscle tightness and muscle weakness. These problems are not reversed by correcting the work station; the individual simply continues to work incorrectly within the corrected work station. These problems are also not corrected with simple instructions; patients typically do not recognize, and often cannot voluntarily correct, their problematic patterns of muscle use and poor posture. EMG monitoring and biofeedback training provide an effective method for detecting and correcting these problems in conjunction with an appropriate therapeutic exercise program.

A Model for the Development and Perpetuation of Chronic Musculoskeletal Pain

The findings of the studies presented above indicate that there is a high rate of occurrence of a number of objective indicators of poor posture and muscle overuse in the area of pain in patients with

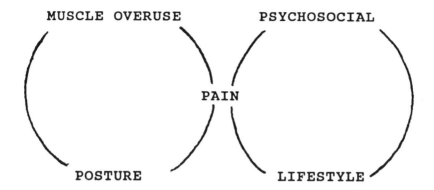

FIGURE 3.10 Dual aspects of chronic myofascial pain: all of these factors can potentially initiate and/or maintain pain and all can interact.

chronic cervical/shoulder girdle pain or chronic headache. The question now becomes, precisely *how* does posture and muscle overuse lead to the development of chronic musculoskeletal pain? The answer probably lies with the following associated factors: localized muscle fatigue, mechanical overload of muscle and joint structures, and muscle imbalances in length and strength that alter complex patterns of muscle use for posture and movement. These factors are potent instigators and perpetuators of musculoskeletal pain.

Figure 3.10 presents a simple conceptual model for the development and perpetuation of chronic musculoskeletal pain. Muscle overuse and posture (left circle) are considered to be relatively direct contributors with effects that are targeted to specific muscles or muscle groups. In contrast, psychological and life-style factors (right circle) are considered to be relatively indirect, with effects that tend to be more diffuse. Each of these can function either as a *risk factor*, which, if faulty, can make the individual more susceptible to chronic musculoskeletal pain (e.g., poor posture), or as a *protective factor* which, if optimal, can render the individual less susceptible to pain problems (e.g., good posture). These factors interact with one another, and this interaction implies that there will seldom be a clear cut one-to-one correspondence between a single factor and problematic pain; rather, the probability of chronic musculoskeletal pain will be increased by the presence of each risk factor and decreased with the presence of each protective factor. For example, Griegel-Morris, Larson, Mueller-Klaus, and Oatis (1992) found that not every individual with severe forward head posture or rounded shoulders reported appreciable cervical/shoulder girdle pain or headache; however, as a group, those with substantial postural deviations reported a significantly higher incidence of musculoskeletal pain and headache than a comparison group with lesser postural problems. The interactive nature of these factors also indicates that treatment programs designed to prevent or remediate chronic musculoskeletal pain would do well to assess, and optimize, each of these factors (Flor, Fydrich, & Turk, 1992).

With this conceptual framework in mind, what do we know about the possible physiological mechanisms through which these factors, particularly muscle overuse and poor posture, produce or perpetuate musculoskeletal pain? The left-hand circle in Figure 3.6 emphasizes that muscle overuse, posture, and musculoskeletal pain are highly interrelated; that each of these three factors can be considered a potential starting point that can foster the development of the other two; and that the interaction between all three can be a potent impetus to the development and perpetuation of chronic pain.

Musculoskeletal Pain

Musculoskeletal pain itself can be a starting point that leads to abnormal posture and muscle overuse. A traumatic injury that produces pain in the muscles and associated connective tissue, for example, will often lead to the development of antalgic (literally, "against pain") postures and protective muscle contractions (bracing and guarding) throughout the area of injury. These are short term strategies (e.g., limping, sitting on one hip, standing bent over) that are designed to protect an acutely injured area by limiting use until healing occurs, and they are often initiated by normal protective reactions to injury, pain, and fear of pain (Hanna, 1988; Kraus, 1988). These strategies are also promoted by voluntary behavior: the individual rapidly learns that pain is minimized by holding the body in an abnormal posture or by avoiding movement. The result may be altered ways of walking, standing, sitting and performing daily activities. While such strategies can be effective over the short term for managing and minimizing acute pain, they foster major problems when continued long term: the abnormal postures and altered patterns of muscle use become habitual and are further reinforced by gradual changes in muscle length, strength, and endurance (Janda, 1988; Kendall, McCreary, & Provance, 1993). These altered postures and patterns of muscle use can be potent sources of continued pain as described below.

Posture

Posture can also be a critical starting point for musculoskeletal pain and muscle overuse. Forward head posture, for example, produces a substantial mechanical stress on the joints of the cervical spine, particularly at the points of connection with the cranium and with the thoracic spine. The weight of the head is now displaced forward of the center of gravity rather than balanced in a normal, gravity-neutral position, and this substantially alters and redistributes the effective mechanical load on the joints and the surrounding connective tissue. Over time, this can be a substantial factor in degenerative changes in the joints. In addition, as the head moves forward the cranium rocks backward on the cervical spine and this reduces the distance between the occiput and the posterior arch of the C1 vertebra. The narrowing of this space and the resulting compression of suboccipital structures has been cited as important in posterior occipital headache (Rocabado, 1983). Postural changes also alter the work loads of the muscles which stabilize and move the effected joints (Fig. 3.7) (Boyd, 1987; Kraus, 1988).

Forward head posture is also associated with rounded shoulders, with mouth breathing, and with increased use of accessory muscles of respiration. As the head shifts forward, it is followed by the upper thoracic spine. This leads to rounded shoulders and a compressed, tight rib cage, with shortened pectoral muscles and reduced chest expansion during respiration. This in turn promotes a shallow, rapid breathing pattern (Darnell, 1983; Kendall et al., 1993; Kraus, 1988). The respiratory effects of forward head posture and rounded shoulders are particularly interesting. Both postures promote overuse of accessory muscles of respiration that include many of the anterior and lateral cervical muscles, such as the clavicular portion of the upper trapezius. These accessory muscles are not designed for continuous respiration but are intended to provide relatively short-term assistance, as, for example, during periods of heavy exertion. Thoracic (as opposed to diaphragmatic) breathing results in a high muscle workload and poor ventilation. Rapid, shallow breathing patterns can decrease PCO_2 and precipitate borderline hyperventilation, with widespread physiological effects that include vasoconstriction, decreased ability to bind and use O_2, and increased nerve and muscle irritability (Fried, 1987). It is therefore not surprising that the mean respiratory rate for the 35 headache patients discussed above (Table 3.1) was 18 breaths per minute and that 36% of these patients had respiratory rates of 20 breaths per minute (bpm) or more. This is in contrast to the 12–16 bpm range that is considered normal: only 51% of headache patients were within this range. Instruction in diaphragmatic breathing is an important part of pain management programs to restore normal respiratory patterns, but instruction needs to be combined with techniques for correcting posture and reducing habitual overuse of accessory muscles of respiration.

The effects of forward head and associated rounded shoulders can be summarized as producing: (1) increased mechanical load on joints; (2) altered patterns of muscle use, and (3) inefficient breathing patterns with a tendency toward hyperventilation. Each of these three factors is an important contributor to musculoskeletal pain. Two recent studies, in addition to those presented in this chapter, support a strong link between posture and pain in the head, neck, and shoulder girdle area. Braun (1991) has reported that women with long-standing temporomandibular pain or dysfunction accompanied by daily headache or cervical pain had a significantly greater mean forward head posture compared with asymptomatic women. In addition, there were differences in two AROM measurements (scapular protraction and retraction) that indicated rounded shoulders and anterior chest wall tightness in the symptomatic group. As noted earlier in this chapter, Griegel-Morris et al. (1992) have reported a higher incidence of cervical and shoulder girdle pain and headache in individuals with pronounced forward head deviations and rounded shoulders.

Posture is, of course, a result of genetic factors such as body dimensions and body composition as well as environmental factors such as imitation of parents' posture, occupation, and choice of leisure activities. Posture can be improved, but if poor posture is long-standing, change can require a systematic postural retraining program that includes therapeutic exercises to stretch tight muscles and strengthen weak muscles: habit retraining with techniques to increase postural awareness; and changes in maladaptive patterns of voluntary muscle used during work and leisure activities.

Muscle Overuse

Muscle overuse can also be a starting point for musculoskeletal pain. There appear to be two major routes through which muscle overuse leads to muscle pain: (1) localized muscle fatigue that is related to muscle circulation and metabolism, and (2) mechanical overload of the muscle that is produced by contractions that exceed the muscle's typical range of generated tension, velocity, or working length. In addition, muscle overuse can cause posture changes by producing muscle tightness, which in turn can alter joint position and motion. Also, overuse of one muscle or muscle group invariably results in underuse of another and so leads to imbalances in muscle length and strength, which can have major postural consequences (Janda, 1988; Kraus, 1988).

Localized Muscle Fatigue

The vast majority of our muscles are intended to be used on an intermittent basis. Even seemingly continuous activities are normally carried out at the level of the muscle through a sequence of alternating contract/relax cycles that provide for circulatory resupply of the working muscle and removal of accumulating metabolic byproducts. For example, the low-back muscles of a normal individual with good posture may show what appears to be a low-level continuous contraction during standing, particularly when EMG signals are averaged over time. However, a close look at the raw EMG signal usually reveals that the muscles are actually repeatedly contracting and relaxing as the person sways slightly forward and backward of his center of gravity (postural sway).

It takes a surprisingly short period of time and a relatively low level of effort to fatigue a muscle that must contract continuously. Objective signs of localized muscle fatigue have been reported for the upper trapezius and supraspinatus muscles within 1 to 5 minutes of continuous muscle contraction at 11% of maximum voluntary contraction (MVC) as indicated by two widely used EMG measures of localized muscle fatigue: increases in mean voltage amplitude (MVA) and decreases in mean power frequency (MPF) (Chaffin, 1973; Hagberg, 1981a; Soderberg, 1992). Others have reported development of fatigue with 5% MVC when the task required one hour of continuous contraction (Jorgenson, Falletin, Krogh-Lund, & Jensen, 1988). In contrast, if the work task alternates contractions with micropauses as short as 2 seconds, endurance time and work capacity are substantially increased (Hagberg, 1981b; Hagberg, 1986).

There is a well-recognized interaction between muscle overuse, localized muscle fatigue, and pain (Enoka & Stuart, 1992; Hagberg & Kvarnstrom, 1984; Klein, Snyder-Mackler, Roy, & De Luca, 1991; Mills, Newham, & Edwards, 1989; Roy, De Luca, & Casavant, 1989). Localized muscle fatigue is accompanied by depletion of muscle energy stores, accumulation of metabolic byproducts, alteration of metabolic processes, and relative ischemia within the muscle. As this process continues, the accumulating metabolites stimulate chemoreceptive pain receptors within the muscle to lower pain thresholds and/or produce pain. This process is greatly accelerated and amplified when a *previously fatigued* muscle is called on to *repeat* a fatiguing activity before the muscle is able to recover its prefatigue state, a process that can take a substantial period of time after the physical activity ends (Broberg & Sahlin, 1989).

It is relevant, therefore, that Hagberg and Kvarnstrom (1984) have reported shorter endurance times for chronically painful muscles (the upper trapezius and supraspinatus muscles on one side of the body) as compared with the same, contralateral, nonpainful muscles of the same subjects. These decreases in endurance appeared to be due to increased fatigability in the painful muscles (rather than the presence of pain), as indicated by corresponding changes in EMG indexes of localized muscle fatigue (increasing MVA and decreasing MPF). Biering-Sorensen (1984) has also found that poor isometric endurance of low-back muscles was a predictor of initial low-back problems over the course of one year following testing. Recent investigations of localized muscle fatigue and low-back pain have reported differences in one or more EMG parameters of muscle fatigue based on EMG power spectral analysis: initial MPF, decline in MPF, and percent of recovery of initial MPF. Differences on one or more of these measures have been found for comparisons of chronic low back pain patients versus normal pain-free individuals (Roy et al., 1989) and for comparisons of varsity athletes with low-back pain versus athletes in the same sport without low-back pain (Klein et al., 1991; Roy, De Luca, Snyder-Mackler, Emley, Crenshaw, & Lyons, 1990). These investigators conclude that fatigue-related measures hold considerable promise as a method for correctly classifying individuals with and without back pain, for determining individuals at particular risk of developing low-back pain, and for investigating the effectiveness of therapeutic exercise regimens for treating low-back pain (Thompson & Biedermann, 1991). At present, it appears that measures of *recovery from fatigue* are particularly promising.

Mechanical Overload of Working Muscle

A second, very common source of musculoskeletal pain is postexertional pain. This is localized muscle pain that is related to heavy or unaccustomed exercise of that muscle, has a delayed onset (often 1 or 2 days after the period of exertion), and may persist for days. It is thought to be related to the amount of mechanical tension generated within the contracting muscle. Muscle contractions that produce delayed-onset pain also cause considerable muscle damage at the ultrastructure level, as indicated by damage to myofibrillar protein structure, disruption of microcirculation, and associated changes in biochemical and radioisotope measures of muscle processes related to injury and repair (Armstrong, Ogilvie, & Schwane, 1983; Mills et al., 1989; Yunis & Kalyan-Raman, 1989). These changes within the muscle can persist 10 days to 3 weeks in normal individuals and far outlast the period of pain. Repeated heavy exertion within that period can carry an added risk.

Several aspects of postexertional pain are particularly relevant to muscle overuse and chronic musculoskeletal pain. Muscle contractions need not be exceptionally strong to produce postexertional pain but need only exceed the muscle's *accustomed* range of generated tension, velocity, or working length. For some normal individuals, this range may be quite small. A muscle that is used for only a narrow range of activities at relatively low generated tensions can experience postexertional pain following activities that require relatively modest tension levels. For many patients with chronically painful muscles and exceptionally low activity levels, this range is likely to be exceeded by the demands of many common daily activities, particularly if these activities are carried out with poor posture and poor body mechanics. In addition, a muscle that is fatigued is at added risk of mechanical overload because of temporary changes within the fatigued muscle, such as slowed contraction time, slowed relaxation time, and reduced elasticity of muscle fibers.

When both muscle fatigue and mechanical overload are considered, there are a number of implications for evaluation and treatment of muscle overuse in individuals with chronic musculoskeletal pain.

1. The individual may perform a task with a stronger contraction than is required due to habitual maladaptive patterns of muscle use. Investigators have noted decreases in circulation in contracting muscle at 10–20% of MVC, with an end result of lowered pain threshold (Hagberg, 1984; Klug, McAuley & Clark, 1989). If the individual uses 20% MVC to perform a task that requires only 5% MVC, this constitutes overuse that can promote premature muscle fatigue. Our experience with chronic pain patients and headache patients performing upper extremity tasks such as computer keyboard operation suggests that this is a very common situation and indicates (Fig. 3.4) that such overuse can lead to rapid development of localized muscle fatigue even in normal pain-free individuals with good activity tolerance.

2. The individual may perform a task using muscles that were not designed for the job. In this case, even low-level tasks may exceed the muscle's strength or endurance capacity. An example here is the use of the cervical muscles for long-term, high-rate respiration, although these muscles are designed for temporary respiratory use. Again, our experience with EMG, recording from cervical muscles, and the high respiratory rates we have documented in many patients with cervical or headache pain indicate that this is a common problem. A second example is use of the suboccipital muscles to support the head in the forward head position.

3. The individual may habitually contract muscles for extended periods of time when no contraction is in fact required, inducing localized muscle fatigue or increasing susceptibility to fatigue when called on to use the muscle for a subsequent high-demand task. Examples here are our data indicating continuous contractions of the upper trapezius muscle while sitting quietly and delayed relaxation following brief voluntary contractions. Slowed muscle relaxation may be related to muscle fatigue and muscle tightness as well as learned factors such as voluntary guarding against movement-induced pain. Delayed relaxation is especially problematic, since it effectively eliminates the "rest" portion of many normal work/rest cycles and is, therefore, highly likely to exacerbate fatigue.

In any case, an overused, easily fatigued, tight muscle is at considerable risk of injury and pain with any sudden increase in demand, whether encountered in ordinary daily activities or in a traumatic event, such as an automobile accident or a fall. The upper trapezius ms, along with the deeper levator scapulae ms, are at particular risk, since they are widely included in numerous activities involving use of the head or the hand. These muscles are also attached, anatomically, to highly mobile skeletal structures such as the occiput, the upper cervical vertebrae, and the scapula, which makes them particularly susceptible to mechanical strain. It is not surprising that these muscles are a common site of pain and trigger points (Hubbard & Berkoff, 1993; Janda, 1988; Middaugh & Garwood, 1989; Travell, & Simons, 1983).

Psychological and Lifestyle Factors

Discussion of the numerous relevant psychological and life-style factors (the right-hand side of the model presented in Fig. 3.10) is well outside the scope of this chapter. However, it is relevant to point out that such factors can have a pronounced, and relatively direct, impact on physiological mechanisms of musculoskeletal pain. For example, low aerobic fitness and disturbed sleep patterns are two factors that are thought to play a major role in development and/or maintenance of chronic musculoskeletal pain (Bennett, Clark, Campbell, & Burckhardt, 1992; Bennett & Goldenberg; 1989). A number of studies have demonstrated that the startle response can briefly produce tightened abdominal muscles, altered breathing patterns, and a protective body posture that includes braced shoulder muscles and forward head (Hanna, 1988; Jones, Hanson, & Grey, 1964). Smoking has been associated with an increased incidence of back pain, possibly due to the vasoconstrictive effects of nicotine or simply as an indicant of reduced fitness or less healthy life-style (Bigos, et al., 1992).

The role of multiple factors in musculoskeletal pain and the strong interaction between physical and psychosocial variables is particularly evident in a recent study by Bigos et al. (1992), who reported on a large prospective study of predictors of acute low-back pain reports in industrial workers. Both physical and psychosocial factors were found to be predictive, including: (1) a medical history of previous back pain (physician visits for back pain in the previous two years) and back pain present during physical examination (back or leg pain with straight leg raise), (2) low job satisfaction (by questionnaire), and (3) elevated MMPI scale 3 (HYSTERIA) indicating distress. It is, therefore, not surprising that there is an accumulating body of evidence linking the sympathetic nervous system to localized muscle fatigue (Seals & Enoka, 1989) and localized muscle pain (Hubbard & Berkoff, 1993; McNulty, Gevirtz, Hubbard, & Berkoff, 1994).

In conclusion, this chapter has highlighted poor posture and muscle overuse as important factors in the development and maintenance of musculoskeletal pain, with data and examples drawn from studies of cervical/shoulder girdle pain and headache. At the same time, as illustrated in Fig. 3.10, these factors are only part of the equation that must be considered, particularly with chronic musculoskeletal pain.

Acknowledgment

This research was supported in part by NIDRR grant No. H133G90085, Department of Education, DHEW, and by the Medical University of South Carolina General Clinical Research Center, NIH grant No. RR1070.

References

Aaras, A., Westgaard, R. H., & Stranden, E. (1988). Postural angles as an indicator of postural load and muscular injury in occupational work situations. *Ergonomics, 31*, 915–933.

Alund, M., & Larsson, S. (1990). Three-dimensional analysis of neck motion: A clinical method. *Spine, 15*, 87–91.

Armstrong, R. B., Ogilvie, R. W., & Schwane, J. A. (1983). Eccentric exercise-induced injury to rat skeletal muscle. *Journal of Applied Physiology, 54*, 80–93.

Arndt, R. (1983). Working posture and musculoskeletal problems of video display terminal operators—review and reappraisal. *American Industrial Hyqiene Association Journal, 44*, 437–446.

Barker, G., & Sellers, A. (1991). *Alteration in Upper Trapezius and Sub-Occipital Muscle Activity Due to Postural Positioning as Measured by EMG*. Master's thesis, College of Health-Related Sciences, Medical University of South Carolina.

Basmajian, J. V. & De Luca, C. J. (1985). *Muscles alive*. Baltimore: Williams & Wilkins.

Bennett, R. M., Clark, S. R., Campbell, S. M., & Burckhardt, C. S. (1992). Low levels of somatomedin C in patients with the fibromyalgia syndrome: A possible link between sleep and muscle pain. *Arthritis and Rheumatism, 35*, 1113–1116.

Bennett, R. M., & Goldenberg, D. L. (Eds.) (1989). *Rheumatic disease clinics of North America: The fibromyalgia syndrome* (Vol. 15, pp. 1–191).

Biering-Sorensen, F. (1984). Physical measurements as risk indicators for low-back trouble over a one-year period. *Spine, 9*, 106–119.

Bigos, S. J., Battie, M. C., Spengler, D. M., Fisher, L. D., Fordyce, W. E., Hansson, T., Nachemson, A. L., & Zeh, J. (1992). A longitudinal, prospective study of industrial back injury reporting. *Clinical Orthopaedic and Related Research, 279*, 21–34.

Boyd, C. H. (1987). The effect of head position on electromyographic evaluations of representative mandibular positioning muscle groups. *The Journal of Craniomandibular Practice, 5*, 50–53.

Braun, B. L. (1991). Postural differences between asymptomatic men and women and and craniofacial pain patients. *Archives of Physical Medicine and Rehabilitation, 72*, 653–656.

Broberg, S., & Sahlin, K. (1989). Adenine nucleotide degradation in human skeletal muscle during prolonged exercise. *Journal of Applied Physiology, 67*, 116–122.

Chaffin, D. B. (1973). Localized muscle fatigue—definition and measurement. *Journal of Occupational Medicine, 15*, 346–354.

Corlett, N., Wilson, J., & Manenica, I. (1985). *The ergonomics of working postures. The proceedings of the first international occupational ergonomics symposium, Zadar, Yugoslavia*. London: Taylor & Francis, 1986.

Cunningham, L. S., & Kelsey, J. L. (1984). Epidemiology of musculoskeletal impairments and associated disability. *American Journal of Public Health, 74,* 574–579.

Darrell, M. W. (1983). A proposed chronology of events for forward head posture. *The Journal of Craniomandibular Practice, 1,* 49–54.

Enoka, R. M., & Stuart, D. G. (1992). Neurobiology of Muscle Fatigue. *Journal of Applied Physiology, 72,* 1631–1648.

Flor, H., Fydrich, T., & Turk, D. C. (1992). Efficacy of multidisciplinary pain treatment centers: A meta-analytic review. *Pain, 49,* 221–230.

Fried, R. (1987). *The hyperventilation syndrome.* Baltimore: Johns Hopkins University Press.

Frymoyer, J. W., & Cats-Baril, W. L. (1991). An overview of the incidence and costs of low back pain. *Orthopedic Clinics of North America, 22,* 263–271.

Griegel-Morris, P., Larson, K., Mueller-Klaus, K., & Oatis, C. A. (1992). Incidence of common postural abnormalities in the cervical, shoulder, and thoracic regions and their association with pain in two age groups of healthy subjects. *Physical Therapy, 72,* 425–431.

Hagberg, M., & Kvarnstrom, S. (1984). Muscular endurance and electromyographic fatigue in myofascial shoulder pain. *Archives of Physical Medicine and Rehabilitation, 65,* 522–525.

Hagberg, M. (1981a). Electromyographic signs of shoulder muscular fatigue in two elevated arm positions. *American Journal of Physical Medicine, 60*(3), 11–121.

Hagberg, M., & Wegman, D. H. (1987). Prevalence rates and odds ratios of shoulder-neck diseases in different occupational groups. *British Journal of Industrial Medicine, 44,* 602–610.

Hagberg, M. (1981b). Muscular endurance and surface electromyogram in isometric and dynamic exercise. *Journal of Applied Physiology, 51*(1), 1–7.

Hagberg, M. (1984). Occupational musculoskeletal stress disorders of the neck and shoulder: A review of possible pathophysiology. *International Archives of Occupational and Environmental Health, 53,* 269–278.

Hagberg, M. (1986). Optimizing occupational muscular stress of the neck and shoulder. In N. Corlett, J. Wilson, & I. Manenica (Eds.), *Ergonomics of working postures* (pp. 109-114). London: Taylor & Francis.

Hanna, T. (1988). *Somatics.* Reading, MA: Addison-Wesley.

Hebert, L. A. (1990). Cumulative trauma prevention. *Clinical Management, 10,* 30–34.

Horowitz, J. M. (1992, October 12). Crippled by computers. *Time* (pp. 70–72).

Hubbard, D. R., & Berkoff, G. M. (1993). Myofascial trigger points show spontaneous needle EMG activity. *Spine, 18,* 1803–1807.

Janda, V. (1988). Muscles and cervicogenic pain syndromes. In R. Grant, (Ed.), *Physical therapy of the cervical and thoracic spine* (pp. 153–166). New York: Churchill Livingstone.

Jones, F., Hanson, J., & Gray, F. (1964). Startle as a paradigm of malposture. *Perceptual Motor Skills, 19,* 21–2.

Jorgenson, K., Falletin, N., Krogh-Lund, C., & Jensen, B. (1988). Electromyography and fatigue during prolonged low-level static contractions. *European Journal of Applied Physiology, 57,* 316–321.

Kantrowitz, B., & Crandall, R. (1990, August 20). Casualties of the keyboard. *Newsweek* (p. 57).

Kasdan, M. L. (Ed.) (1991). *Occupational hand and upper extremity injuries and diseases.* Philadelphia: Hanley & Belfus.

Kellett, K. M., Kellett, D. A., & Nordholm, L. A. (1991). Effects of an exercise program on sick leave due to back pain. *Physical Therapy, 71,* 283–293.

Kendall, F. P., McCreary, E. K., & Provance, P. G. (1993). *Muscles, testing and function: With posture and pain* (4th ed). Baltimore: Williams & Wilkins.

Kilbom, A., Persson, J., & Jonsson, B. (1985). Risk factors for work-related disorders of the neck and shoulder—with special emphasis on working postures and movements. In N. Corlett, J. Wilson, & I. Manenica (Eds.), *Erqonomics of workinq postures* (pp. 44–53). London: Taylor & Francis.

Klein, A. B., Snyder-Mackler, L., Roy, S. H., & De Luca, C. J. (1991). Comparison of spinal mobility and isometric trunk extensor forces with electromyographic spectral analysis in identifying low back pain. *Physical Therapy, 71,* 445–453.

Klug, G. A., McAuley, E., & Clark, S. (1989). Factors influencing the development and maintenance of aerobic fitness: Lessons applicable to the fibrositis syndrome. *Journal of Rheumatology, 16* (Supplement 19), 30–39.

Kraus, S. S. (1988). Cervical spine influences on the craniomandibular region. In S. L. Kraus (Ed.), *TMJ disorders: Management of the craniomandibular complex* (pp. 367–404). New York: Churchill Livingstone.

McNulty, W., Gevirtz, R., Hubbard, D., & Berkoff, G. (in press). Needle electromyographic evaluation of trigger point response to a psychological stressor. *Psychophysiology.*

Middaugh, S., & Kee, W. G. (1987). Advances in electromyographic monitoring and biofeedback in treatment of chronic cervical and low back pain. In M. G. Eisenberg & R. C. Grzesiak (Eds.), *Advances in clinical rehabilitation,* vol. 1. New York: Springer Publishing Co.

Middaugh, S. J. (1992). A muscle physiology approach to mechanisms and treatment of chronic musculoskeletal pain. *Symposium on mechanisms and treatment of chronic muscle pain: Current theories and evidence, 23rd annual meeting of the association for applied psychophysiology and biofeedback,* March 19–24, Colorado Springs.

Middaugh, S. J. (1989). Biobehavioral Techniques. In R. Scully & M. Barnes (Eds.), *Physical therapy* (pp. 986–997). Philadelphia: Lippincott.

Middaugh, S. J., & Garwood, M. K. (1989). A new approach to the key muscle hypothesis. *Proceedings of the association for applied psychophysiology and biofeedback, 20th annual meeting* (pp. 145–148).

Middaugh, S. J., Woods, S. E., Kee, W. G., Harden, R. N., & Peters, J. R. (1991). Biofeedback-assisted relaxation training for chronic pain in the aging. *Biofeedback and Self-Regulation, 16,* 361–377.

Millender, L. H., Louis, D. L., & Simmons, B. P. (Eds.) (1992). *Occupational disorders of the upper extremity.* New York: Churchill Livingstone.

Mills, K. R., Newham, D. J., & Edwards, R. H. T. (1989). Muscle pain. In P. Wall & R. Melzack (Eds.), *Textbook of pain.* New York: Churchill Livingstone.

Onishi, N., Nomura, H., & Sakai, F. (1973). Fatigue and strength of upper limb muscles of flight reservation system operators. *Journal of Human Ergonomics, 2,* 133–141.

Putz-Anderson, V. (Ed.) (1988). *Cumulative trauma disorders: A manual for musculoskeletal diseases of the upper limbs (NIOSH).* New York: Taylor & Francis.

Raab, D. M., Agre, J. C., McAdam, M., & Smith, E. L. (1988). Light resistance and stretching exercise in elderly women: Effect upon flexibility. *Archives of Physical Medicine and Rehabilitation, 69,* 268–272.

Rocabado, M. (1983). Biomechanical relationship of the cranial, cervical and hyoid regions. *The Journal of Craniomandibular Practice, 1,* 61–66.

Roy, S. H., De Luca, C. J., Snyder-Mackler, L., Emley, M. S., Crenshaw, R. L., & Lyons, J. P. (1990). Fatigue, recovery, and low back pain in varsity rowers. *Medicine and Science in Sports and Exercise,* 463–469.

Roy, S. H., De Luca, C. J., & Casavant, D. A. (1989). Lumbar muscle fatigue and chronic lower back pain. *Spine, 14,* 992–1001.

Seals, D. R., & Enoka, R. M. (1989). Sympathetic activation is associated with increases in EMG during fatiguing exercise. *Journal of Applied Physiology, 66,* 88–95.

Smith, M. J., Cohen, B. G. F., Stammerjohn, Jr., L. W., & Happ, A. (1981). An investigation of health complaints and job stress in video display operations. *Human Factors, 23,* 387–400.

Smith, M. J., Stammerjohn, L. W., Cohen, B. G. F., & Lalich, N. R. (1980). Job stress in video display operations. In E. Grandjean & B. Vigliani (Eds.), *Ergonomic aspects of visual display terminals* (pp. 201–210). London: Taylor & Francis.

Soderberg, G. L. (Ed.) (1992). *Selected topics in surface electromyography for use in the occupational setting: Expert perspectives,* DHHS (NIOSH) Publication No. 91-100. Washington, DC: NIOSH.

Sternbach, R. A. (1986). Survey of pain in the United States: The Nuprin Pain Report. *Clinical Journal of Pain, 2,* 49–53.

Thompson, D. A., & Biedermann, H. J. (1991). Sensitivity of electromyographic spectrum analysis of paraspinal muscles to changes following physical training. *Rehabilitation R & D Progress Reports* (pp. 236–237), Washington, DC: VHSRA.

Travell, J. C., & Simons, D. G. (1983). *Myofascial pain and dysfunction: The trigger point manual.* Baltimore: Williams and Wilkins.

Youdas, J. W., Carey, J. R., & Garrett, T. R. (1991). Reliability of measurements of cervical spine range of motion—comparison of three methods. *Physical Therapy, 71,* 98–106.

Youdas, J. W., Garrett, T. R., Suman, V. J., Bodard, C. L., Hallman, H. O., & Carey, J. R. (1992). Normal range of motion of the cervical spine: An initial goniometric study. *Physical Therapy, 72,* 770–780.

Yunis, M. B., & Kalyan-Raman, U. P. (1989). Muscle biopsy findings in primary fibromyalgia and other forms of nonarticular rheumatism. In R. M. Bennett & D. L. Goldenberg (Eds.), *Rheumatic disease clinics of North America: The fibromyalgia syndrome, Vol. 15* (pp. 115–134). Philadelphia: Saunders Co.

Chapter Four

Pain Proneness in Children: Toward a New Conceptual Framework

Julie E. Goodman, Yori Gidron, and
Patrick J. McGrath

This chapter will examine psychological risk factors that contribute to the development and maintenance of chronic and recurrent pain problems during childhood or adolescence. Although there are some data on the childhood risk factors that are pertinent in the development of a chronic pain condition during adulthood, our focus will be limited to the discussion of childhood and adolescent pain problems.

What does Psychological Vulnerability Mean?

The first step in examining the concept of psychological vulnerability to chronic pain is to explore the meaning of the construct. What exactly does it mean to say that a child is psychologically vulnerable, pain prone, or at greater psychological risk of developing and/or maintaining a pain problem? There are a number of possible meanings. For example, such a child could show one or more of the following risks: an increased risk of having any type of pain; an increased risk of having a specific type of pain; an increased risk of having pain of unknown origin; an increased risk of psychologically caused pain; a heightened sensitivity to pain (either lower threshold or increased symptom reporting); an increased risk of displaying pain behaviors; an increased risk of showing an exaggerated response to pain; or an increased risk of serious interference with social roles because of pain (i.e., a social handicap).

It is important to differentiate among these types of pain proneness because different mechanisms might be operative for each. Typically, a global nonspecific construct of pain proneness has been used that has resulted in confusion regarding the precise meaning of this concept. The mechanisms underlying pain proneness have received scant attention in the literature. Moreover, there are varying levels of research support for the occurrence of the different types of pain proneness. For example, there is a relatively large body of research regarding the contribution of psychological factors to the development of recurrent abdominal pain in children, whereas very little research has investigated the risk factors of developing a pain-related handicap secondary to recurrent abdominal pain. Finally, reference is rarely made to a theoretical framework around which new and existing data can be interpreted to clarify the nature of various types of pain proneness.

The World Health Organization (WHO, 1980) model of the impact of chronic diseases provides a conceptual framework which has been adapted for pain (McGrath, Mathews, & Pigeon, 1990). The WHO model proposes four "planes of experience" through which the impact of pain on an individual can be interpreted: underlying cause, impairment, disability, and handicap. The underlying cause refers to the physiological or psychological cause of the pain. Impairment refers to the manifestation of the underlying cause, most commonly seen as pain symptoms. Disability refers to the interference with or disruption of specific activities as a result of pain. Finally, handicap is the interference with social roles because of pain. Although different planes of experience may influence each other, there is not necessarily a uniform relationship among the planes. For example, two children with the same underlying problem and even the same levels of pain could have very different levels of handicap.

Using the WHO model, increased risk for pain could occur within any of the four planes of experience: increased risk of having the underlying cause for a pain condition (e.g., the physiological substrate of migraine); increased risk for experiencing pain as a symptom (e.g., headache); increased risk for pain-related disability (e.g., difficulty doing school work during attacks); or increased risk

TABLE 4.1 Hypothetical Model of Pain Proneness in Migraine

Type of Pain Proneness	Source of Pain Proneness			
	Disease Factors	Family Factors	Individual Factors	Psychosocial Factors
Underlying Cause	spreading cortical depression	family stress	depression, anxiety	adolescent predilection to skip breakfast

for pain-related handicap (e.g., school failure). There also could be multiple sources of a single type of pain proneness. Table 4.1 illustrates how there could be different sources of pain proneness for the underlying cause of migraine. Pain proneness can occur as a result of disease factors, factors within the individual, family factors, or sociocultural factors. For example, in terms of the underlying cause of migraine, pain proneness could be due to a risk of spreading cortical depression or serotonin dysfunction. In addition, risk factors for the underlying cause of migraine could also include depression, anxiety, or family stress.

The four different types of pain proneness and their different sources can be combined to form a matrix. The rows of the matrix indicate the type of pain proneness and columns represent the sources of pain proneness. Table 4.2 outlines how such a matrix could describe the different planes of experience for recurrent abdominal pain.

Because the goal of this chapter is to examine the psychological factors that affect pain proneness, the focus will be on the psychological factors within the individual, within the family, and within a social and/or cultural realm, and spend little time directly discussing physiological and disease factors. To more effectively organize the literature, the issues pertaining to family and individual factors will be discussed according to pain condition and, where possible, findings of research will be discussed in terms of the WHO model.

Recurrent Abdominal Pain

Recurrent abdominal pain is a common childhood problem. Apley and Naish (1958) defined recurrent abdominal pain as pain with no identifiable organic cause that recurs at least three times during a 3-month period and interferes with activities. They estimated that this pain

TABLE 4.2 Hypothetical Model of Pain Proneness in Recurrent
Abdominal Pain

Type of Pain Proneness	Source of Pain Proneness			
	Disease Factors	Family Factors	Individual Factors	Psychosocial
Underlying Cause	*	inherited tendency to abdominal pain	depression, anxiety	low fiber in diet
Pain as a Symptom	*	familial exaggeration of pain	low pain threshold	cultural acceptance of pain complaints
Pain-related disability	*	modelling of sports avoidance	anxiety, depression	expectation to be passive when ill
Pain-related handicap	*	modelling, reinforcement	encouragement of sick role for abdominal pain	

*by definnition, the underlying organic cause of recurrent abdominal pain is not known (Apley, 1958).

problem affects approximately 10% of children, although the incidence changes dramatically depending on the age and sex of the child.
There is considerable disagreement regarding which psychological
factors, if any, are implicated in the etiology and maintenance of recurrent abdominal pain. The following section will describe evidence
pertaining to specific psychological factors and their relationship to
the etiology of recurrent abdominal pain. There will also be an attempt to discuss the psychological risk factors associated with developing a pain-related disability or handicap resulting from recurrent
abdominal pain; however, there has been very little attention directed
to this aspect of recurrent abdominal pain in the literature.

Underlying Cause of Recurrent Abdominal Pain

By definition, the etiology of recurrent abdominal pain is unknown. This is a central obstacle to making inferences about how

psychological factors affect the physiological bases. Nevertheless, there is considerable research in this area (e.g., Apley & Naish, 1958; Zuckerman, Stevenson, & Bailey, 1987).

Family Factors

Several reports have noted the tendency of recurrent abdominal pain patients to come from families with a positive family history of recurrent abdominal pain and other painful disorders that are often accompanied by emotional disturbance and anxiety (e.g., Apley & Naish, 1958; Hughes & Zimin, 1978; Zuckerman, Stevenson, & Bailey, 1987). In addition, there are no sound epidemiological studies that clearly demonstrate aggregation of recurrent abdominal pain in families (Goodman & McGrath, 1991). The simple aggregation of similar pain problems among family members is not sufficient evidence to suggest that family factors play a causal role in their etiology and does not account for the contribution of constitutional similarities within family members to the occurrence of recurrent abdominal pain.

A controlled study by McGrath, Goodman, Firestone, Shipman, and Peters (1983) compared children with recurrent abdominal pain (defined according to Apley's 1975 criteria) to a control group of children attending outpatient clinics for minor health problems and their families with the intent of examining a number of psychological variables believed to be associated with psychogenicity. Although the recurrent abdominal pain group reported more pain symptoms as preschoolers (abdominal pain and other pain symptoms), the two groups showed no difference in the frequency with which their parents and siblings reported pain symptoms. This finding counters the common assertion that children with recurrent abdominal pain come from families who experience more pain. As well, the study did not identify any family variables that could account for a child developing recurrent abdominal pain, as no group differences were found on measures of marital adjustment or life change.

The findings of Walker and Greene (1989) suggested that maternal anxiety plays a role in the development of recurrent abdominal pain. Mothers of children with recurrent abdominal pain showed higher levels of anxiety, depression, and somatization than mothers of control children. Although the study could not determine that the mothers' distress level was not a reaction to their child's disorder, it was concluded that maternal distress was likely implicated in the development and maintenance of recurrent abdominal pain.

In another study, Walker, Garber, and Greene (1991) showed that higher levels of somatization in parents were associated with higher levels of somatization in children with recurrent abdominal pain but not in children with organically based abdominal pain or in control children. These findings are also suggestive of parental modeling through which recurrent abdominal pain can develop.

Somatization in relatives of children with recurrent abdominal pain was also the focus of investigation in a study by Routh and Ernst (1984). Recurrent abdominal pain was defined as abdominal pain occurring in the absence of a medical diagnosis for more than 1-year prior to the medical examination of the study. The incidence of somatization disorder in first- and second-degree biological relatives of children with recurrent abdominal pain was compared to those with organically based abdominal pain. Fifty percent of children with recurrent abdominal pain were found to have relatives with somatization disorder, whereas only 5% of children with organically based abdominal pain were found to have relatives with somatization disorder. Ernst, Routh, and Harper (1984) hypothesized that recurrent abdominal pain may be a precursor to adult somatization disorder. However, the authors did not explore the meaning of the link between somatization disorder and recurrent abdominal pain other than suggesting a common genetic predisposition to developing "hysterical" symptoms within families, even though there was no evidence that the recurrent abdominal pain symptoms in their sample were "hysterical" in nature. Further, relatives identified with somatization disorder were not questioned whether they had experienced recurrent abdominal pain during childhood. It is unclear whether a direct link exists between the two disorders. It appears that the recurrent abdominal pain group had more direct and indirect exposure to somatization than did the group with organically based abdominal pain. Modeling of pain behavior also appears to be a plausible psychological mechanism through which somatization disorder could be linked to recurrent abdominal pain, but this mechanism was not mentioned.

A study by Hodges, Kline, Barbero, and Woodruff (1985) reported that a more direct link between parental anxiety, child anxiety, and the etiology of recurrent abdominal pain may exist. In this study, children with recurrent abdominal pain and their parents were identified as having more anxiety than healthy controls, but similar levels of anxiety when compared to children with behavior problems and their parents. The authors speculated that, in the recurrent abdominal pain group, increased levels of anxiety could trigger a reactive gastrointestinal tract that could cause symptoms of recurrent abdominal pain. Parents and children who had similar levels of anxiety but who did not show symptoms of recurrent abdominal pain may not have a reactive gastrointestinal tract. Data from the same sample showed that mothers of children with recurrent abdominal pain reported more depressive symptoms than mothers of healthy children but that children with recurrent abdominal pain did not report more depressive symptoms than healthy controls (Hodges et al., 1985). Because children with recurrent abdominal pain may be more anxious than healthy controls (Hodges et al., 1985), they may react more adversely to a parent's depressive symptomatology, which may, in turn, exacerbate their pain condition.

Individual factors

Apley (1975) noted that recurrent abdominal pain may be a response to stress from family or school problems among anxious, socially unskilled, and self-conscious children. However, these views were based more on clinical impressions than empirical findings.

McGrath, Goodman, Firestone, Shipman, and Peters (1983) found no significant differences between children with recurrent abdominal pain and pain-free controls on measures of depression and personality. This study questioned the validity of the traditional "psychogenic" profile typically implied in recurrent abdominal pain in that no direct link between psychological factors and pain could be identified.

Attempting to address the issue of causality, Sawyer, Davidson, Goodwin, and Crettenden (1987) compared children with recurrent abdominal pain to children with organically based abdominal pain and pain-free controls on measures of emotional and behavioral problems. The organic group showed more internalizing behavior (as rated by mothers) than the two other groups, and the recurrent abdominal pain group was rated as significantly more sociable. These findings run counter to the description offered in Apley (1975), which portrays the child with recurrent abdominal pain as anxious and socially unskilled. Teachers rated children with recurrent abdominal pain as more psychologically disturbed than healthy children as measured on the Rutter B2 Behavioral Scale. There was no significant difference between the children with recurrent abdominal pain and children with organically based pain on this measure.

Comparing children and adolescents with recurrent abdominal pain, organically based abdominal pain, and healthy controls, Walker and Greene (1991b) found no significant differences between the groups on the number of stressful events occurring during the previous year. However, there was a significant relationship between negative life events and pain at a 3-month follow-up for children with recurrent abdominal pain. Those children with recurrent abdominal pain who reported fewer negative life events were more likely to show symptom resolution than were those who had initially reported more negative life events. Further, among recurrent abdominal pain patients, negative life events occurring subsequent to the initial clinic visit predicted somatization and anxiety at follow-up. The authors suggested that biological mechanisms such as intestinal motility could be affected by the stress of negative life events or that such negative events could affect the course of recurrent abdominal pain by interfering with the ability to cope with the syndrome.

Using parental reports, Wasserman, Whitington, and Rivary (1988) showed no differences between recurrent abdominal pain and healthy children regarding negative life events occurring within the previous 3 months. These results and those of Walker and Greene (1991b) are inconsistent with the earlier findings of Hodges, Kline, Barbero, and Flanery (1984), who found that children with recurrent abdominal pain and behaviorally disordered children reported significantly more negative life events in the previous year than healthy controls. However, in all three of the aforementioned studies, the temporal relation between the development of recurrent abdominal pain and the occurrence of negative life events was not investigated. Studies using prospective designs would facilitate our understanding of these possible relationships.

Psychosocial Factors

Dimson (1971) found that children with recurrent abdominal pain had a slower transit time than did controls suggesting that they might become constipated more easily. A randomized clinical trial of treatment of recurrent abdominal pain with dietary fiber supplements supported the view that constipation might cause the pain (Feldman, McGrath, Hodgson, Ritter, & Shipman, 1985). Consequently, life-style or cultural factors that promote a low-fiber diet might trigger abdominal pain in susceptible individuals.

Although the physiological basis of recurrent abdominal pain is unknown, it is believed that psychological variables could play a role in its etiology. The previous studies all examined psychological factors that may affect the onset and maintenance of recurrent abdominal pain in children. By examining the psychological correlates of this pain problem, it is hoped that the mechanism underlying recurrent abdominal pain will be better understood. The following section will examine studies that focus primarily on psychological factors that affect the frequency with which children report or complain of recurrent abdominal pain.

Symptom Reporting

Reporting pain as a symptom is a type of pain behavior that communicates to others that one is experiencing pain and discomfort. There is considerable evidence that pain behaviors, including symptom reporting, can be reinforced by means of operant conditioning and can be extinguished using simple behavioral techniques (Fordyce, 1976).

Family Factors

Miller and Kratochwill (1979) provided an excellent example of how reinforcement of symptom reporting can occur within the context of the family. A 10-year-old girl had been reporting severe abdominal pain daily for over a year. After each pain complaint, her mother would administer medication, require her to rest, and provide her with books, toys, and access to television. The episodes typically lasted between 30 minutes and 3 hours, during which the girl would make requests for food, drinks, and attention. Her mother typically fulfilled all of her requests and provided her with constant attention. The frequency of the child's complaints were reduced to 1 per month using a simple time-out procedure that was designed to eliminate excessive social attention (e.g., TV, toys, visits on demand from her mother), while continuing to acknowledge her pain with rest and administering medication. This reduction was maintained at a 1-year follow-up. It is unclear whether the reduction in symptom reporting was indicative of a reduction in the patient's experience of pain. However, it does appear that the procedure was extremely successful in reducing the extent of pain-related disability and handicap (e.g., school absence), which was associated with pretreatment levels of symptom reporting.

Opportunities for children to learn about pain are seemingly endless. Children are routinely exposed to their own and other children's everyday pain experiences, such as the bumps and bruises incurred during childhood play (Fearon, McGrath, & Achat, personal communication; Craig, 1983), but the precise nature of the learning processes involved are poorly understood.

There is conflicting evidence regarding the extent to which children learn about pain from salient models such as parental figures. Walker and Greene (1989) suggested that children could learn illness behavior as a coping strategy via the process of modeling of maternal somatization. However, as other authors have noted, it has not yet been firmly established that recurrent abdominal pain occurs more frequently in children from "pain-prone" families where the opportunity for observing pain behavior would be relatively high (Lavigne, Schulein, & Hahn, 1986). A child's report of pain and/or their coping strategies for pain may be more responsive to psychological factors such as modeling than is the underlying cause of pain (McGrath & Unruh, 1987, p. 153).

Relatively recent research provides evidence that recurrent pain problems in children may be related to the family environment of the child. For example, Osborne, Hatcher and Richtsmeier (1989) examined the role of social modeling of pain and illness behavior in unexplained pediatric pain. Children referred to a tertiary care facility with either recurrent abdominal or recurrent chest pain with no known organic etiology were compared to children with recurrent pain secondary to sickle-cell disease on the number of models of pain and illness behavior in the child's environment. Comparisons were also done on the parents of the children in both groups. An interview was used to assess the location, intensity, frequency, and environmental consequences of the children's and models' pain. Referred children with unexplained pain were more likely to identify a model of pain or illness behavior than were children with explained pain. These findings suggest that children with recurrent unexplained pain may come from what Apley (1975) has called a "painful family," in which there is a greater likelihood of a child being exposed to a salient person displaying pain and illness behavior. The group of children with unexplained pain and their models were more likely to report positive or neutral consequences of their pain, whereas children with explained pain were more likely to report negative consequences. These findings suggest that the social environment of the child may contribute to the maintenance of symptom reporting. However, similar factors may concurrently contribute to the development of the pain problem or to the associated disability and handicap. Further research is needed to clarify the nature of these relations.

Individual Factors

Walker and Greene (1989) found that children with recurrent abdominal pain and those with organically based abdominal pain reported significantly higher levels of depression, trait-anxiety, somatization, and pain compared to healthy controls but did not differ from each other. Increased anxiety, depression, and somatization were found in both the recurrent abdominal pain group and the organically based abdominal pain group, which suggests that this profile may result from having a painful syndrome; however, this is speculative. High levels of somatization were observed again at the 3-month follow-up in children with recurrent abdominal pain. The authors believed that children with recurrent abdominal pain were less likely to experience symptom resolution as a result of medical intervention as compared to those children with organically based abdominal pain (Walker & Greene, 1989).

Walker and Greene (1991b) suggested that negative events may affect the prognosis and symptom dimensions of recurrent abdominal pain. It is not clear whether the occurrence of negative life events is more related to the maintenance of recurrent abdominal pain as a syndrome (i.e., pain and disability) or whether they affect symptom reporting, or both.

Psychosocial Factors

There is no information pertaining to how psychosocial factors such as peer influence or cross-cultural differences might influence symptom reporting in recurrent abdominal pain. It is clear that cultural differences contribute to the pain response (e.g., Fritz, Schechter, & Berstein, 1991), but these differences are poorly understood.

Pain-Related Disability and Handicap

Apley's diagnostic criteria for recurrent abdominal pain stipulates that pain-related disability and/or handicap, defined as interference with the child's activities, must accompany the cluster of presenting symptoms to be considered a case of recurrent abdominal pain.

Family Factors

Very little is known about the extent to which family factors such as parental modeling or encouragement of illness and/or pain behavior impact on the extent of disability and handicap exhibited by children with recurrent abdominal pain, as no systematic research has been conducted in this area. Walker and Zeeman (1992) recently reported on the development of a self-report instrument, the Illness Behavior Encouragement Scale, designed to measure parental responses to child illness behavior. This instrument will likely facilitate research that will help to identify the parental factors and other psychological factors that may contribute to the development of illness behavior that could promote and discourage disability and handicap.

Individual Factors

Daily activities have often been used as a proxy measure of disability and handicap resulting from chronic pain in adults (e.g., Skevington, 1983). The Functional Disability Inventory (Walker &

Greene, 1991a) is a relatively new instrument that was developed to assess the extent to which activities of daily living in children are disrupted as a result of physical health. Although not specifically designed for use with pain, preliminary research with this instrument (e.g., Gidron, McGrath, & Goodday, 1992) has shown that it can be used as a measure of the disability and handicap related to postoperative pain. The Functional Disability Inventory will likely facilitate research that will contribute to our understanding of how psychological factors are related to the development and maintenance of pain-related disability and handicap in children.

Psychosocial Factors

No research has been conducted that examines how psychosocial factors are related to disability and handicap secondary to recurrent abdominal pain.

Comment

Certain psychological constructs such as depression or somatization may empirically and theoretically overlap with some of the planes of experience as outlined in the WHO model. For example, it is often difficult to distinguish between the social aspects of depression and pain-related handicap; avoidance or withdrawn from social activities could be viewed as either a symptom of depression or part of a pain-related handicap. It is important to examine the context surrounding symptoms whose origin or etiology is not readily apparent. If a child is avoiding activities because of pain, it would be appropriate to consider this symptom as part of a pain-related handicap. If a child is avoiding activities because they are feeling sad, it would be appropriate to consider depression. If scores on measures of depression and pain-related handicap are both elevated, it may be a result of item redundancy in the measures being used.

Another concern with research on recurrent abdominal pain is one of generalizability. Most of the research regarding recurrent abdominal pain uses patients selected from tertiary-care clinics. Children who meet the criteria for recurrent abdominal pain who are referred to a tertiary-care clinic may be quite different and/or may have family members who are quite different from those children who meet the criteria for recurrent abdominal pain but who are not referred. It may be that parental anxiety plays a role in the referral of children with recurrent abdominal pain for medical examination (Walker & Greene, 1989), rather than contributing directly to the onset of symptoms.

Headache and Migraine

The classification system developed by the International Headache Society (IHS, 1988) outlines 12 different types of headache disorders, cranial neuralgias, and facial pain; each type has several different subtypes. This classification system provides more specific and detailed criteria for headache, which allows more reliable and consistent diagnoses. It classifies types of headache rather than types of headache sufferers. This classification system was developed only recently. Thus, little systematic research has been conducted on how psychological factors may affect or influence the onset of well-defined specific types of headache. Furthermore, a recurrent headache sufferer is likely to have more than one type of headache, and the types of headache a patient has may change considerably over time (McGrath & Unruh, in press). That headache is such a complicated disorder creates problems for conducting research and when interpreting existing data.

Underlying Cause of Headache

Unfortunately, the basic nature of migraine and tension-type headache are poorly understood. For a more in depth discussion of these factors, please see *The Headaches*, edited by Oleson, Tfelt-Hansen, and Welch (in press).

Family Factors

The most consistent finding in research on headache and migraine is that a headache sufferer is likely to show a positive family history for the disorder. Traditional methods of diagnosing migraine incorporate the identification of a parent who suffers from migraine as part of the diagnostic criteria. This practice undoubtedly reduces the significance of aggregation of migraine within the family because cases of migraine-like symptoms not showing a positive family history would not be classified as migraine. Thus, knowledge of aggregation would contribute little to identifying any common mechanisms responsible for the development of migraine in children and their parents (McGrath & Unruh, in press).

There has been some suggestion that a mother's psychological state, particularly maternal depression and/or anxiety, is implicated in the development and onset of headache and migraine in children (Zuckerman, Stevenson, & Bailey, 1987). The majority of studies attempting to document this relationship have either shown evidence of serious methodological difficulties or have failed to delineate the nature of the mechanisms involved in maintaining the relationship.

Individual Factors

Bille (1962) compared children who had "pronounced migraine" occurring at least once a month and pain-free controls. Parental reports revealed that the migraine group was more anxious, sensitive, had less self-control, and was more tidy than controls. Children with migraine, particularly girls, described themselves as more anxious, fearful, and tense than controls. Finally, 60% of the children with migraine (significantly more girls) continued to have migraines in adulthood. These findings imply that high levels of anxiety in childhood may increase the risk for chronic migraine later in life, particularly in women.

Andrasik, Kabela, Quinn, Attanasio, Blanchard, and Rosenblum (1988) found that children with migraine reported significantly more symptoms of depression and somatization than non-headache peer-matched controls. Male adolescents with migraine were significantly more anxious and showed poorer overall psychological adjustment compared to controls. Although the two previously mentioned studies included pain-free controls, it cannot be inferred whether the elevations noted on the psychological measures were a cause or a result of headache.

Attempting to address this question, Cunningham, et al. (1987) compared a group of children with migraine to a group of "pain controls" (children with musculoskeletal pain) and "no pain" controls on several standardized psychosocial measures. The three groups did not differ significantly on measures of anxiety or depression, with the exception of teachers reporting the headache group to show significantly more anxiety than the two control groups. Parental reports revealed that children with headaches showed significantly less social competence and reported more somatic complaints than both control groups. It was also noted that anxiety, depression, somatization, and personality variables significantly correlated with pain severity. However, after controlling for pain severity, the three groups did not differ significantly on any of the psychological variables, with the exception of the headache group scoring significantly higher on migraine-related somatic complaints. It appears that the psychological characteristics often associated with childhood migraine are common to other chronic pain syndromes. In addition, because controlling for pain severity eliminated most differences observed between groups, it may be that elevated scores on certain psychological measures (e.g., anxiety, depression, somatization) may be a result, rather than a cause, of recurrent or chronic pain.

Additional support for the link between anxiety and migraine comes from an uncontrolled intervention study which found that initial low levels of trait anxiety significantly predicted reductions of headache frequency and intensity in children and adolescents with recurrent headaches (Smith, Womac, & Chen, 1990). Depression did not predict either of these reductions, and was significantly lower following reductions in headache frequencies. However, this study did not have a control group and did not provide data on the initial correlation between anxiety and depression.

Taken together, the above studies show a mixed picture regarding psychological factors and headache. There is some empirical support for the notion that anxiety may be implicated in the cause of migraine, which may then precipitate depressive episodes. It has also been suggested that life interferences resulting from migraine can lead to disability and reduced perceived self-control, which also may precipitate depression (Rudy, Kearns, & Turk, 1988). With respect to the planes of experience outlined in the WHO model (McGrath, Mathews, & Pigeon, 1990), anxiety may alter an individual's pain threshold or tolerance (France, Krishnan, & Houpt, 1988) and contribute to reporting more headache symptoms. Depression may be associated with the dimensions of disability and handicap (Rudy, Kearns, & Turk, 1988).

The contribution of stress and negative life events to the onset of headache and migraine have also been the subject of investigation. Passchier and Orlebeke (1985) reported that 30–40% of children experiencing headache at least once a month cited stress as the primary precipitating factor. However, "stress" was never clearly defined in their discussion, and it is not known whether the authors' operational definition was provided for the children prior to the time when they gave their responses.

Andrasik et al. (1988) found no differences between children and adolescents with recurrent migraine and matched controls on a score of life change in the last 6 months. In an uncontrolled adult intervention trial with three types of chronic headache groups, life changes in the last year or 6 months did not predict reduced headache intensity (Blanchard et al., 1983). According to a few relatively sound studies, it appears that negative life events are not related to headache severity. Further studies with reliable and valid assessment instruments are needed in this area.

Psychosocial Factors

There are no data on how psychosocial factors may contribute to the underlying cause of migraine.

Other Types of Pain Proneness

There is very little data on how family, individual, or psychosocial factors affect symptom reporting and disability and handicap in headache and migraine. The WHO framework, as applied to pain proneness, can be used to direct future research in these areas.

Dysmenorrhea

Dysmenorrhea is defined as painful menstruation usually occurring on the first and second day of menstruation, characterized by cramping pain in the lower abdomen and often accompanied by nausea, vomiting, edema, and headache (Klein & Litt, 1981; Holmlund, 1990). It is important to note that dysmenorrhea is distinct from what has been termed "premenstrual syndrome," which, by definition, precedes menstruation and refers to a variety of physical and psychological symptoms (Holmlund, 1990).

Underlying Cause

Family Factors

Although there are some data on how maternal modeling and encouragement of menstrual symptoms impacts on the adult experience of dysmenorrhea (Whitehead, Busch, Heller, & Costa, 1986), there is very little research that examines these relations during childhood and adolescence.

Individual Factors

Klein and Litt (1981) investigated the effect of "preparation for menarche" on the occurrence of dysmenorrhea or subsequent school absence but found no significant effects. Preparation was defined as whether the subject was informed about what menstruation was prior to menarche and was assessed using a single-item retrospective scale. Postmenarcheal age accounted for the greatest proportion of variance in the occurrence of dysmenorrhea, with younger women reporting dysmenorrhea less often than older women.

Psychosocial Factors

There is quite an extensive body of literature suggesting that the symptoms associated with dysmennorhea are related to culturally induced beliefs and stereotypes. For example, Brooks-Gunn and Ruble (1982) showed that negative beliefs and stereotypes about menstruation were related to more severe menstrual symptoms in a sample of girls aged 11–14 years. Although the development of menstrual-related beliefs in girls is not yet well understood, it may be that altering these beliefs could alter symptom severity.

Other Types of Pain Proneness

There are very little data available on how family, individual, or psychosocial factors affect symptom reporting and disability and handicap associated with dysmennorhea during adolescence. Only one study has been conducted in this area. In a prospective study, Holmlund (1990) examined personality variables at age 15 and the experience of primary dysmenorrhea (i.e., without pelvic abnormalities) at age 25 in a nonclinical sample of 349 adolescents. The author concluded that no personality differences existed between women who experience dysmenorrhea and those who do not. However, women with severe dysmenorrhea, defined as experiencing handicap in several areas of functioning, reported higher levels of guilt at both ages than controls without dysmenorrhea at both ages. Holmlund also suggested that adolescents with severe dysmenorrhea at age 15 showed less self-confidence than women who never experienced dysmenorrhea but compensated for this by being more achievement oriented and aggressive at age 25. These findings are somewhat surprising given that, when compared to women who never experienced dysmenorrhea, women with severe dysmenorrhea reported that they were more conventionally feminine, a trait which appears to be inconsistent with being aggressive and achievement oriented.

Other Types of Pain

Disability and Handicap

Family and Individual Factors

Dunn-Geier, McGrath, Rourke, Latter, and D'Astous (1986) examined the differences between adolescents who had a chronic or recurrent pain condition (either knee pain, stomachaches, or headaches), who were coping well with their pain, and those who were not coping well (i.e., those who were missing school) on measures of mother–child interaction, child personality, and family characteristics. No group differences were found on measures of pain intensity or duration obtained using a daily pain diary. Noncoping adolescents engaged in more negative behavior and expressed more pain than coping adolescents during the experimental tasks, which consisted of exercises designed to simulate typical daily activities that may cause pain. Mothers of noncoping adolescents were observed as discouraging coping behavior during these tasks more frequently and were significantly more involved with their children's participation. No differences were found between the two groups on measures of personality or general family environment. This study suggested that pain-related disability may be related to parental responses to adolescents' pain behavior.

Similar findings were reported in a study by Varni, Thompson-Wilcox, Hanson, and Brik (1988). A number of psychological variables believed to have a negative impact on the functional status of children with chronic musculoskeletal pain resulting from juvenile rheumatoid arthritis were the subject of investigation. Results showed that child psychological adjustment, as measured by the internalizing and externalizing dimensions on the Child Behavior Checklist, family psychosocial environment, as measured by the Family Environment Scale (FEE), and pain status, as measured by the Varni/Thompson Pediatric Pain Questionnaire (PPQ), statistically predicted scores on the Child Activities of Daily Living Index. These initial findings suggested that there may be an interactive relationship between pain status, pain-related disability, and certain psychological variables, including family functioning and the psychological functioning of the child. Studies of this nature have important implications for assisting health care professionals in predicting who might be at risk for developing more severe levels of pain and pain-related disability in children who have a chronic painful condition.

Children of Chronic Pain Patients

There is considerable evidence that chronic pain in adults can disrupt normal family functioning. The emphasis of this body of research is on the psychological distress and marital dissatisfaction experienced by the spouses of patients when the husband is the identified patient (for reviews, see Turk, Flor, & Rudy, 1987a; Payne & Norfleet, 1986). Parental chronic pain may also have a negative impact on the children in that family (e.g., Richard, 1988). Craig (1983) has suggested that parents can serve as models of pain behavior for children, which may influence the expression of pain behavior in children. Further, there is some indication that the prevalence of pain problems in the families of adult chronic pain patients is significantly higher than in the general population

(Violon & Giurgea, 1984), and that there exists a positive relation between the number of "pain models" in an individual's family environment and the frequency of their pain complaints (Edwards, Zeichner, Cuczmierczyk, & Boczkowski, 1985). However, the mechanisms underlying these relationships have not been thoroughly investigated, and the ages when these relationships begin to develop and exert the most influence are not known.

A study by Rickard (1988) noted that children whose fathers had chronic low back pain exhibited a higher frequency of behaviors hypothesized to have been learned by observing and interacting with parental chronic pain behaviors than children of either healthy controls or diabetic parents. These behaviors were assessed by asking children to respond to hypothetical scenarios depicting situations in which pain behaviors or a variety of other behaviors could be emitted. Children of chronic low-back pain patients also showed higher levels of teacher-rated conduct problems and behavior problems than the children in the other two groups. Modeling of abnormal illness behavior by chronic pain patients was cited as a possible explanation of how children could have developed this symptom profile.

Raphael, Dohrenwend, and Marbach (1990) showed that women with temporomandibular pain and dysfunction syndrome reported higher frequencies of illnesses in their children over a 10-month period than did healthy controls. Although these differences could be attributed to a reporting bias in the women with chronic pain, there were no differences in the frequency with which the two groups reported illnesses and injuries in their spouses and in other important people. However, the authors did not provide information regarding whether the higher levels of illness were a result of specific diseases or disorders or whether they reflected general somatic complaints. This study provides evidence that children of women with a chronic pain syndrome may be at risk for experiencing illness more frequently than are their counterparts; however, the authors were unable to examine the mechanisms underlying how this occurs.

Dura and Beck (1988) examined multiple aspects of family functioning in the families of mothers with either chronic pain, a chronic illness (diabetes), or no illness. Although children of mothers who had chronic pain reported higher levels of depressive symptomatology than did children in the other groups, the authors did not examine how chronic pain in a parent might affect the frequency of pain complaints and physical symptom reporting in children.

It is clear that research examining the impact of parental chronic pain on children is only beginning to address the large number of factors that may be implicated in the development and maintenance of chronic or recurrent pain problems in children. There is presently considerable empirical support that parental modeling of illness behavior is one of the psychological mechanisms involved in the development of recurrent or chronic pain in children; however, it is not yet known on which factors (e.g., symptom reporting, disability, handicap) modeling is likely to have the largest impact.

Summary and Conclusion

Pain proneness in children is not a thoroughly researched area. Most studies have used retrospective methods to examine the psychological correlates of developing a pain problem, rather than directly addressing the issue of pain proneness. For example, are children with recurrent abdominal pain more anxious than children without recurrent abdominal pain? This type of methodology does not permit the researcher to determine whether psychological factors are implicated in the cause of pain or whether they are a result of having pain.

Vulnerability to pain-related disability and handicap is the most poorly understood and researched type of pain proneness. Pain severity is not a reliable predictor of the extent of pain-related disability or handicap, as there is generally no uniform relation between these variables (McGrath, Mathews, & Pigeon, 1991). Further research is necessary to determine whether certain psychological variables, such as parental modeling, or coping style are predictive of disability or handicap.

Future research should also take care to avoid the methodological pitfalls of previous studies. Problems of sampling biases, inconsistent operational definitions of pain syndromes, and reliability and validity of measurements all affect the overall utility of a particular study. Furthermore, very little attention has been paid to cross-cultural differences in the etiology and impact of pain syndromes. These factors must be addressed before we can begin to piece together a more meaningful picture of how psychological factors can increase or decrease the likelihood of developing a chronic or recurrent pain problem during childhood.

References

Andrasik, F., Kabela, E., Quinn, S., Attanasio, V., Blanchard, E. B., & Rosenblum, E. L. (1988). Psychological functioning of children who have recurrent migraine. *Pain, 34,* 43–52.

Apley, J. (1975). *The Child with abdominal pain* (2nd ed.). Oxford: Blackwell Scientific.

Apley, J., & Naish, N. (1958). Children with recurrent abdominal pains: A field survey of 1000 school children. *Archives of Disease in Childhood, 33,* 165–170.

Bible, B. (1962). Migraine in schoolchildren. *Acta Pediatrica Scandinavia Supplement, 51,,* 1–151.

Blanchard, E. B., Andrasik, F., Arena, J. G., Neff, D. F., Jurish, S. E., Teders, S. J., Barron, K. D., & Rodichok, L. D. (1983). Nonpharmacologic treatment of chronic headache: Prediction of outcome. *Neurology, 33,* 1596–1603.

Brooks-Gunn, J., & Ruble, D. N. (1982). The development of menstrual-related beliefs and behaviors during early adolescence. *Child Development, 53,* 1567–1577.

Cunningham, S. J., McGrath, P. J., Ferguson, H. B., Humphreys, P., D'Astous, J., Latter, J., Goodman, J. T., & Firestone, P. (1987). Personality and behavioural characteristics in pediatric migraine. *Headache, 27,* 16–20.

Craig, K. D. (1983). Modeling and social learning factors in chronic pain. In J. J. Bonica et al. (Eds.), *Advances in pain research and therapy, vol. 5* (pp. 813–827). New York: Raven.

Dimson, S. B. (1971). Transit time related to clinical findings in children with recurrent abdominal pain. *Pediatrics, 47,* 666–674.

Dunn-Geier, B. J., McGrath, P. J., Rourke, B. P., Latter, J., & D'Astous, J. (1986). Adolescent chronic pain: The ability to cope. *Pain, 26,* 23–32.

Dura, J. R., & Beck, S. J. (1988). A comparison of family functioning when mothers have chronic pain. *Pain, 35,* 79–89.

Edwards, P., Zeichner, A., Kuczmierczyk, A., & Boczkowski, J. (1985). Familial pain models: The relationship between family history of pain and current pain experience, *Pain, 21,* 379–384.

Ernst, A. R., Routh, D. K., & Harper, D. C. (1984). Abdominal pain in children and symptoms of somatization disorder. *Journal of Pediatric Psychology, 9,* 77–86.

Feldman, W., McGrath, P. J., Hodgson, C., Ritter, H., & Shipman, R. T. (1985).

The use of dietary fibre in the management of simple idiopathic recurrent abdominal pain: Results in a prospective double-blind randomized controlled trial. *American Journal of Diseases of Children, 139,* 1216–1218.

Fordyce, W. E. (1976). *Behavioral methods for chronic pain and illness.* St. Louis: CV Mosby.

France, R. D., Krishnan, K. R. R., & Houpt, J. L. (1988). Overview. In R. D. France & K. R. R. Krishnan (Eds.), *Chronic pain,* Washington DC: American Psychiatric Press.

Fritz, K. I., Schechter, N., & Bernstein, B. (1991). Cultural components of pain behavior in Vietnamese refugee children. *Journal of Pain and Symptom Manaqement, 6*(3), 205.

Gidron, Y., McGrath, P. J., & Goodday, R. (1992). The psychosocial and physical predictors of physical and functional recovery from oral surgery in adolescents. Presented at the 5th International Congress of *The Pain Clinic,* Jerusalem, Israel.

Goodman, J. E., & McGrath, P. J. (1991). The epidemiology of pain in children and adolescents: A review. *Pain, 46,* 247–264.

Hodges, K., Kline, J. J., Barbero, G., & Flanery, R. (1984). Life events occurring in families of children with recurrent abdominal pain. *Journal of Psychosomatic Research, 28,* 185–188.

Hodges, K., Kline, J. J., Barbero, G., & Flanery, R. (1985). Depressive symptoms in children with recurrent abdominal pain and in their families. *Journal of Pediatrics, 107*(4), 622–626.

Hodges, K., Kline, J. J., Barbero, G., & Woodruff, C. (1985). Anxiety in children with recurrent abdominal pain and their parents. *Psychosomatics, 26*(11), 859–866.

Holmlund, U. (1990). The experience of dysmenorrhea and its relationship to personality variables. *Acta Psychiatrica Scandinavia, 82,* 182–187.

Hughes, M. C., & Zimin, R. (1978). Children with psychogenic abdominal pain and their families. *Clinical Pediatrics, 17*(7), 569–573.

Klein, J. R., & Litt, I. F. (1981). Epidemiology of adolescent dysmenorrhea. *Pediatrics, 68,* 661–664.

Lavigne, J. V., Schulein, M. J., & Hahn, Y. S. (1986). Psychological aspects of painful medical conditions in children. II. Personality factors, family characteristics and treatment. *Pain, 27,* 147–169.

McGrath, P. J., Goodman, J. T., Firestone, P., Shipman, R., & Peters, S. (1983). Recurrent abdominal pain: A psychogenic disorder? *Archives of Disease in Childhood, 58,* 888–890.

McGrath P. J., Mathews, J., & Pigeon, H. (1990). Assessment of pain in children. In M. R. Bond, J. E. Charlton, & C. J. Woolk (Eds.), *Pain research and clinical management, vol. 4, proceedings of the VI world congress on pain* (pp. 509–526). Amsterdam: Elsevier.

McGrath, P. J., & Unruh, A. M. (1987). *Pain in children and adolescents.* Amsterdam: Elsevier.

McGrath, P. J., & Unruh, A. (in press). *Pain in children and adolescents* (2nd ed.). Amsterdam: Elsevier.

Miller, A. J., & Kratochwill, T. R. (1979). Reduction of frequent stomachache complaints by time-out. *Behavior Therapy, 10*, 211–218.

Oleson, J., Tfelt-Hansen, P., & Welch, K. M. A. (in press). *The headaches*. New York: Raven.

Osbourne, R. B., Hatcher, J. W., & Richtsmeier, A. J. (1989). The role of social modelling in unexplained pediatric pain. *Journal of Pediatric Psychology, 14*(1), 43–61.

Passschier, J., & Orlebeke, J. F. (1985). Headaches and stress in schoolchildren: An epidemiological study. *Cephalalgia, 5*, 167–176.

Payne, B., & Norfleet, M. A. (1986). Chronic pain and the family: A review. *Pain, 26*, 1–22.

Raphael K. G., Dohrenwend, B. P., & Marbach, J. J. (1990). Illness and injury among children of temporomandibular pain and dysfunction syndrome (TMPDS) patients. *Pain, 40*, 61–64.

Rickard, K. (1988). The occurrence of maladaptive health-related behaviors and teacher-rated conduct problems in children of chronic low back pain patients. *Journal of Behavioral Medicine, 11*(2), 107–116

Routh, D. K., & Ernst, A. R. (1984). Somatization disorder in relatives of children and adolescents with functional abdominal pain. *Journal of Pediatric Psychology, 9*(4), 427–437.

Rudy, T. E., Kerns, R. D., & Turk, D. C. (1988). Chronic pain and depression: Toward a cognitive-behavioral meditation model. *Pain, 35*, 129–140.

Sawyer, M. G., Davidson, G. P., Goodwin, D., & Crettenden, A. D. (1987). Recurrent abdominal pain in childhood. Relationship to psychological adjustment of children and families: A preliminary study. *Australian Paediatric Journal, 23*, 121–124.

Skevington, S. M. (1983). Activities as indices of illness behavior in chronic pain. *Pain, 15*, 295–307.

Smith, M. S., Womac, W. M., & Chen, C. N. (1990). Intrinsic patient variables and outcome in the behavioral treatment of recurrent pediatric headache. *Advances in Pain Research Therapy, 15*, 305–311.

Turk, D. C., Flor, H., & Rudy, T. E. (1987a). Pain and families. I. Etiology, maintenance and psychosocial impact. *Pain, 30*, 3–27.

Violon, A., & Giurgea, D. (1984). Familial models for chronic pain. *Pain, 18*, 199–203.

Walker, S. L., Garber, J., & Greene, J. W. (1991). Somatization symptoms in pediatric abdominal pain patients: Relation to chronicity and parent somatization. *Journal of Abnormal Child Psychology, 19*, 379–394.

Walker, L. A., & Greene, J. W. (1989). Children with recurrent abdominal pain and their parents: More somatic complaints, anxiety, and depression than other patient families? *Journal of Pediatric Psychology, 14*(2), 231–243.

Walker, L. A., & Greene, J. W. (1991a). The functional disability inventory:

Measuring a neglected dimension of child health status. *Journal of Pediatric Psychology, 16*(1), 39–58.

Walker, S. L., & Greene, J. W. (1991b). Negative life events and symptom resolution in pediatric abdominal pain patients. *Journal of Pediatric Psychology, 16,* 341–360.

Walker, L. A., & Zeeman, J. L. (1992). Parental response to child illness behavior. *Journal of Pediatric Psychology, 17*(1), 49–71.

Wasserman, A. L., Whitington, P. F., & Rivary, F. P. (1988). Psychogenic basis for abdominal pain in children and adolescents. *Journal of the American Academy of Child and Adolescent Psychiatry, 27,* 179–184.

Whitehead, W. E., Busch, C. M., Heller, B. R., & Costa, P. T., Jr. (1986). Social learning influences on menstrual symptoms and illness behavior. *Health Psychology, 5*(1), 13–23.

World Health Organization (1980). *International classification of impairments, disabilities, and handicaps.* Geneva: World Health Organization.

Zuckerman, B., Stevenson, J., & Bailey, V. (1987). Stomachaches and headaches in a community sample of preschool children. *Pediatrics, 79*(5), 677–682.

Chapter Five

Chronic Daily Headache and the Elusive Nature of Somatic Awareness

Donald Bakal, Stefan Demjen, and Paul N. Duckro

Chronic daily headache is recognized clinically as the one of the most difficult of the headache disorders to understand and to treat. With this headache, the pain seldom presents as a distinct attack with a definite beginning and end, making it impossible for clinicians to analyze the condition in terms of specific psychological and physical causes or triggers. The headache sufferers themselves, waking as they do with pain already present, cannot fathom what factors external or internal to themselves could possibly be responsible. Overuse of analgesic medication is common and observations of causative or ameliorative factors are often inaccurate. Clearly, the plan for treatment of this headache syndrome must be different from the treatment which is typically used in the management of episodic forms of tension and migraine headache.

The defining characteristic of chronic daily headache is its unremitting or intractable nature. There are no specific sensory or physiological symptoms that can be used to differentiate daily headache from episodic headache variants. The vast majority of chronic daily headaches begin as episodic headaches, and the transition from episodic headache attacks to daily headache generally goes unnoticed by the sufferers themselves. More than 20 headache days per month has been suggested as a criterion for daily or near-daily headache (Wilkinson, 1988).

Although chronic daily headache was only recently recognized as a diagnostic entity, a similar condition was identified by Harold Wolff in his classic studies of migraine sufferers (Ostfeld & Wolff, 1958). In making repeated observations of migraine episodes, Wolff (1937) noticed that the majority of his patients were seldom pain free outside of the migraine attack:

> There is another type of head pain which occurs in migraine patients. It may be present concomitantly or in the interval between migraine attacks. Such headache is nonpulsatile, of low or moderate intensity, and may last for days, weeks, or years. The individual feels as if he has a hat on when he has none; that his neck is in a cast; that his shoulders are sore; that if he could be rubbed he would feel more comfortable. Action potentials recorded from the head and neck muscle during such a headache indicate vigorous contraction. (p. 1503)

Wolff clearly described the essence of the chronic daily headache syndrome but did not view these persistent low-grade symptoms as having import for understanding the etiology of the more dramatic symptoms accompanying migraine attacks. It is not known what percentage of episodic migraine and tension headache sufferers function throughout the night and day with similar low-grade symptoms outside of their actual headache attacks.

The International Classification Committee of the International Headache Society (1988) proposed that the label "chronic tension-type headache" be used instead of chronic daily headache, and that inclusion criteria reflect tension headache symptoms (pressing/tight pain, bilateral, moderate severity) and not migraine symptoms (no vomiting, no more than one migraine symptom). There is no evidence, however, that chronic daily headache is restricted to tension headache symptoms. In fact, we observed in several studies (Bakal, 1982) that both tension and migraine headache symptoms increase in prevalence with increasing hours of experienced head pain. Mathew (1991) described the majority of their clinical cases as beginning with migraine and evolving into daily headache with mixed features of migraine and tension headache. Clinicians have long observed that migraine pain may also become daily in nature, hence the term "status migrainous."

Some specialists believe that prolonged and excessive analgesic medication is the cause of chronic daily headache. Many studies have found that withdrawal of analgesic and other abortive medications is associated with reduction of headache activity (Cantwell-Simmons, Duckro, & Richardson, in press). For example, Diener et al. (1989) followed 139 patients with chronic daily headache who were withdrawn from medications in hospital over a 2-week period. During this period many patients exhibited a number of withdrawal symptoms, which in many instances resembled severe headache symptoms (nausea, vomiting, diarrhea, stiff neck, inability to sleep). At discharge, 45% of the patients were headache free. At a mean 2.9 year follow-up, the improvement rate had dropped considerably, but 66% of the subjects reported some maintained improvement in their chronic headache activity. However, these same subjects continued to use some form of medication, although at levels greatly reduced from those reported prior to hospitalization.

It is difficult to state with certainty what changes lead to improvement in headache following analgesic withdrawal; in most reports drug withdrawal was not done without other supportive treatment. The fear of experiencing even worse pain without analgesic medication is a major component of the general distress of these individuals. Improving following analgesic discontinuation usually occurs in clinical environments and may result from lowered distress levels while in hospital or while receiving new treatment. Thus brief periods of hospitalization and discontinuation of medication are, in many instances, accompanied by subtle alterations in the psychobiologic processes affecting the daily headache. In addition, not all daily headache patients demonstrate daily use of symptomatic medication. For these reasons, it may be premature to label daily headache as "analgesic-induced" headache. Nevertheless, it may often be necessary to withdraw these individuals from their dependence on analgesic medication to break the cycle of daily pain. To have the gains maintained, however, patients must recognize factors other than the medication reduction/change as also critical in their improvement. Without this reduction and associated behavioral treatment, gains will likely be temporary and limited to a "honeymoon" period.

The primary thesis of this chapter is that chronic daily headache needs to be understood and managed from a psychobiological systems perspective, with emphasis on headache-related experiential variables within the sufferers themselves. Hospitalization, removal of analgesics, changes in medication, living arrangement, diet, and so forth can be utilized to break the daily pattern but will not lead to long-term benefits unless accompanied by changes in the patient's awareness of the underlying psychobiological processes.

The Psychobiological Model

Our approach to the study of daily headache has been conducted within the context of a severity or psychobiologic model of headache disorders (Bakal, 1982; Bakal, Demjen, & Kaganov, 1984). Basically, the severity model holds that chronic daily headache reflects the evolution of episodic headache associated with two critical factors: (1) the individual's failure to cope with less severe/frequent headaches, and (2) increasing involvement and automaticity of the underlying psychological and physiological processes. The model proposes that patients with varying episodic headache syndromes share, in part, psychobiologic factors that predispose them to the daily headache syndrome. These factors are both continuous and multifaceted in nature, involving cognitive, behavioral, physiological, and biochemical events.

Other formulations of chronic daily headache recognize the nonspecific evolutionary nature of the condition and suggest that psychiatric or neurologic factors may account for the transformation from episodic tension or migraine headache to the pattern of daily headache. In 1983, Saper, Johnson, and van Meter presented data on a large sample of chronic daily headache sufferers, showing that in all cases their headaches began as an intermittent condition and progressed through changes in unknown mechanisms to a daily pattern. Saper (1988) suggested that the transformation from intermittent headache to daily headache reflected a "spontaneous biological transformation" associated with a central disturbance of neurotransmitter/receptor function. Both depression and substance abuse were seen as possible antecedents of these changes. Olesen (1991) noted that the condition often involves psychological disturbance and drug abuse as well as central supraspinal facilitation and peripheral myofascial and vascular input. The notion of increased central nervous system sensitivity of these individuals is based on demonstrations of decreased pain thresholds, which include regions far from removed from the site of the headache (Schoenen, Gerard, De Pasqua, & Juprelle, 1991).

The notion that tension and migraine headache disorders share some common etiological features is becoming increasingly accepted (Saper, 1988). This recognition will result in a better understanding of the complex psychobiologic processes that lead to the development and maintenance of the chronic daily headache syndrome. Despite the quality of clinical observations that have accumulated in the last decade, there is still a great deal to be learned about the psychobiology of chronic daily headache. Nevertheless, there are in practice definite self-regulatory strategies that can be adapted by patients and clinicians to prevent and manage the condition.

Systemic models are increasingly being used to conceptualize health and illness and are especially useful for conceptualizing the biochemical, physiological, perceptual, cognitive, personality, and interpersonal factors that contribute to headache susceptibility. We present somatic awareness as the critical system parameter, enhancement and utilization of which will ameliorate daily headache. We also explore factors that make somatic awareness such a difficult concept for patients to employ.

Premonitory Warnings

Biobehavioral interventions based on relaxation training and biofeedback require recognizing developing pain early, even to the point of noticing sensory/physiological events that reliably precede pain (Duckro, 1990). Episodic headache sufferers generally have an easier time with this requirement than daily headache sufferers. Most chronic daily headache sufferers, in spite of the pervasiveness of their condition, show a degree of fluctuation in their pain intensity, symptom pattern, and distress levels over a 24–hour period. Quite often they are at their best during the early hours of the day or during the hours immediately preceding sleep. There is nothing in the fluctuating headache activity, however, which strikes the daily sufferer as having preventive or pain-management potential.

The first signs of increasing headache activity and how they are coped with can tell us much about daily headache sufferers. Generally, they ignore the signs of lesser headaches because, in their words, they "can stand the lesser pain." Recognition of early headache activity is perceived as having no coping value, other

TABLE 5.1 Premonitory Headache Symptoms
Experienced On The Day Of Attack (modified from
Amery, Waelkens & Vandenbergh, 1986)

Sensory Symptoms	Affective Symptoms
pallor	depressive feelings
altered facial feelings	taciturn, inactive
blurred vision	crying
photophobia	irritable
nausea	difficulty concentrat-
dizziness	ing
aching muscles	
adynamia	
paresthesias	

than indicating that one must prepare for another period of worsening pain, sickness and disappointment. Why dwell on a condition, they say, which is going to become worse—better to get on with the day as long as one can.

The avoidance of the first signs of headache activity is a common reaction of all headache sufferers. If their attention is directed internally, however, these individuals are able to recognize a number of sensations and lesser pain symptoms that otherwise would have been ignored. Table 5.1, adapted from Amery, Waelkens, and Vandenbergh (1986), lists symptoms reported by migraine patients on the day of their attack. Amery et al. noted that the majority of these symptoms were themselves characteristic of a form of headache. The symptoms in the first column have a sensory quality and signify to the sufferer that his/her developing headache is likely to worsen. The symptoms in the right column have an emotional quality and are often driven by anticipation of pain and suffering, based on the patient's perception of the likelihood of impending severe headache. One area that needs to be explored is the extent to which such symptoms, especially during the development stage, might be utilized by headache sufferers to prevent or abort the actual headache episode. That is, by utilizing the first signs of headache to take effective coping action, it may be possible to prevent the worsening of the condition to a point where self-regulation becomes extremely difficult, if not impossible. Such symptoms are seldom seen in this light.

Amery et al. (1986) documented a number of positive correlations between the reported presence of premonitory symptoms and indices of headache severity: duration of disorder, duration of headache attacks, number of identified trigger factors, number of accompanying symptoms, number of aggravating factors, and number of post-attack symptoms all correlated with the frequency of reported premonitory symptoms. They also observed that it was often difficult to distinguish when a premonitory symptom ended and the headache began, since the same symptoms characterized both states.

Premonitory headache symptoms may have their beginnings during sleep. The vast majority of chronic daily headache sufferers have pain or beginnings of pain present upon awakening. This pattern has been observed in both adults and children (Bakal et al., 1984). Furthermore, there is evidence (Demjen, Bakal & Dunn, 1990) that individuals with daily headache experience a number of significant prodromal symptoms upon awakening, including persistent neck tightness, nausea, and feverlike sensations. The headache-alleviating power of sleep has been known for a long time. In 1863, John Hilton published a classic text titled *Rest and Pain*, with the theme that rest to an injured tissue is essential to its recovery (Walls & Philipp, 1953). It is common knowledge that sleep is the most effective natural means for alleviating acute headache. In fact, headache may have the primary biologic function of signifying tissue fatigue and the need for sleep.

Chronic daily headache sufferers are able to sleep, but they seldom feel rested or restored following a night's sleep. Many will report that they had a good night's sleep and are puzzled with the presence of premonitory and/or pain symptoms upon awakening. A similar nonrestorative sleep pattern was reported by Moldofsky (1989) to characterize a number of musculoskeletal symptoms that fibromyalgia sufferers experience upon awakening. Described as a miserable flu-like feeling, the condition was characterized by headache, generalized muscle aching, loss of appetite, tiredness, nervousness, and irritability.

There are no identified physiologic correlates of nonrestorative sleep in daily headache sufferers. Studies with episodic headache occurring at night have suggested a relationship of onset with REM sleep (Dexter, 1987), but the implications of this observation for clinical treatment are not evident. Muscular hyperactivity is a suspected component of nonrestorative sleep, and yet there is no evidence in support of such an hypothesis. Hatch et al. (1991) required episodic headache sufferers to wear a computer-controlled electromyographic (EMG) activity recorder in their natural environment for 48 to 96 consecutive hours. Although there was a highly significant difference between the mean EMG activity during sleep and that recorded during waking, there was little evidence supporting a relationship between EMG activity and headache onset. They gave an example of one patient who rated neck pain high on retiring and waking, but did not evidence elevated EMG at that site during the night. The absence of EMG activity, however, does not rule out the possibility of underlying muscle irritation.

More research is required for understanding the psychobiological processes that are initiated during sleep and lead to the onset of premonitory headache symptoms. For example, analgesic medications taken for the headache itself could be a factor in the symptoms on waking, with increased headache being generated as the patient withdraws from the medicine. Particular attention needs to be directed to the psychological state of headache sufferers prior to and during sleep. Clinical evidence suggests the presence of considerable anxiety, worry, and depression in these patients, which are likely to disturb sleep in themselves. They report affect-related characteristics such as worry over the headache itself, difficulty feeling comfortable, concern about the day's events, and feeling tense. Depression may also have biochemical effects on sleep quality and pain threshold, whether it is secondary or primary in the clinical presentation. These reports suggest that one component affecting sleep may be the reaction to headache itself.

Waking Thoughts and Coping Styles

The failure of chronic daily headache sufferers to use premonitory sensory information becomes more understandable when one examines the thoughts and feelings that accompany their headache disorder. Their cognitions are not what one might see in the occasional headache sufferer. Demjen, Bakal, & Dunn (1990) developed a headache cognitions questionnaire to examine the thoughts and feelings that take place immediately before and during headache

TABLE 5.2 Headache Cognitions (adapted from Demjen et al., 1990)

1. I am worried about how long this headache will last
2. I am depressed because I have another headache
3. I am angry with myself for getting another headache
4. I can think of nothing other than pain
5. I am wondering why I am getting a headache now
6. How am I going to concentrate with this awful headache
7. I feel frustrated about not being able to control pain
8. I am thinking, "Why me? Why do I always get headaches?"
9. I feel annoyed about petty and irrelevant things
10. I am critical of another person
11. I wish people would be more considerate
12. I have no patience with others

attacks. In daily headache sufferers, the questionnaire is completed in reference to when the pain is least severe and most severe. Factor analysis revealed two interpretable factors, called "headache-related thoughts" and "situation-related thoughts." Sample items from the questionnaire are presented in Table 5.2. Items 1 through 8 represent headache-related thoughts, and items 9 through 12 represent situation-related thoughts.

Patients who reported headache pain for more than 8 hours per day had a greater percentage of headache-related thoughts than episodic headache patients. They were also less likely to view situational stress as a factor that maintains headache. Thus daily headache is accompanied by a cognitive shift in which the headache syndrome itself becomes the dominant focus. These patients may acknowledge stress, but it is attributed to the headache problem rather than to events of everyday life, which are often recognized by episodic patients as independent contributors to headache activity. Many chronic headache patients believe that "if I didn't have the headache, I would be fine." Ignoring situational stressors in favor of the headache pain compounds the plight of these patients.

Specific coping strategies used by headache sufferers to deal with pain have been identified in studies using the Coping Strategies Questionnaire (CSQ; Rosenstiel & Keefe, 1983). The CSQ is a 42–item questionnaire that measures the strategies used by chronic pain patients to cope with pain. There are seven coping dimensions assessed by the questionnaire: (1) diverting attention (thinking of things that serve to distract attention away from the pain), (2) coping self-statements (telling oneself that one can cope with the pain, no matter how bad it gets), (3) ignoring pain sensations (denying that the pain hurts), (4) praying or hoping (telling oneself to hope and pray that the pain will get better someday), (5) increased behavioral activities (engaging in active behaviors that divert one's attention away from the pain), (6) reinterpretation of pain sensation (imagining something that is inconsistent with the experience of pain), and (7) catastrophizing (negative self-statements, catastrophizing thoughts and ideation).

Spinhoven, Jochems, Linssen, and Bogaards (1991) administered the CSQ to 111 chronic tension-headache patients. Factor analysis identified a major factor, accounting for 38% of the variance, which was labeled active coping and consisted of trying to ignore pain, increasing activity, using coping statements, and diverting attention. This factor was positively correlated with duration of pain. Their findings are consistent with clinical reports that suggest that encouraging patients to ignore pain and to push on will only aggravate the situation. Other data has also suggested that although distraction is a frequently used coping strategy and is effective with acute pain of low intensity, it is not effective with intense and or chronic pain (McCaul & Malott, 1984). Chronic or intense pain stimuli are too insistent to be avoided successfully. They bring to mind the adage, "You can run, but you can't hide."

The belief that chronic headache sufferers should ignore their headache pain is held by both practitioners and patients themselves. Philips (1987), for example, described avoidance as the most frequent and maladaptive of coping styles utilized by headache sufferers. Avoidance is defined broadly to include any activity (movement, social interactions, leisure) that the headache sufferer ceases because of the pain. Philips observed that such avoidance behavior seldom has any therapeutic benefit. Philips proposed that the avoidance continues not because of pain but because of negative expectations and beliefs. The negative expectations seen in daily headache sufferers is understandable, given that they begin each day with pain present and have no perceived effective strategies for reducing headache activity, especially in interpersonal situations. Avoiding the underlying sensory/physiological symptoms and putting on a "brave face" for them represents the only alternative, but unfortunately this strategy is usually accompanied by a worsening of their condition. What is required to solve this dilemma is recognition by daily headache sufferers of the negative impact of chosen coping strategies. This recognition can be attained through a greater appreciation by patients of the psychobiological processes that maintain their condition.

Somatic Awareness

The study of preheadache warnings suggested that there may be a "window of opportunity" early in the headache process that might allow the patient to abort or mitigate the worsening headache. As the condition worsens, the probability of successfully lessening the condition diminishes, but the objective remains the same. The goal is to have the headache sufferer use somatic awareness to reduce the likelihood of increased pain or to reduce existing pain. Defining somatic awareness is not a simple matter; as a concept it is rich in "surplus meaning," an advantage in the clinical situation but difficult for teaching. Somatic awareness has been defined by Cioffi (1991) as the process by which we perceive, interpret, and act on the information from our bodies. To be effective, the awareness needs to be accompanied by an alteration of the sensory symptoms. This state is variously described as letting go, the relaxation response, the quieting response, and passive relaxation. The combination of awareness and letting go is quite powerful and if successfully implemented can lead to recovery similar in nature to the recovery associated with restorative sleep.

If one were to characterize the various levels of variables controlling chronic daily headache in terms of levels or layers that needed discovery, then somatic awareness would constitute the core of the discovery process. Although the concept often does not find its way into the conscious treatment plan for headache disorders, it is not a completely novel concept either historically or in nonmedical situations. It seems to be best understood in sports psychology, in which athletes use somatic awareness to enhance performance. Morgan and Pollock (1977) reported more than 15 years ago that elite marathon runners, when compared to their less experienced counterparts, used an associative rather than a dissociative cognitive strategy in dealing with sensations while running. Dissociative strategies had no relation to the sensory experiences of running and included techniques such as recalling early experiences, working mathematical exercises, and hearing favorite music. These strategies were also accompanied by efforts to "run or fight through" the pain when it became noticeable, which led to increased discomfort, pain and discouragement. Elite runners, on the other hand, paid especially close attention to bodily sensations arising in their feet, calves, and chest. They repeatedly reminded themselves to relax and "stay loose" during the run. They also dismissed the marathon concept of "the wall" as myth—they simply did not come up against the wall during the run. Morgan and Pollock (1977) speculated that elite runners are able to associate (monitor) their sensory input and adjust their pace and technique accordingly.

Hanna (1988) coined the term "sensory-motor amnesia" (SMA) to describe the lack of somatic awareness that characterizes individuals with chronic pain problems:

> For example, while a client with a chronically sore shoulder is lying on my padded work table, I lift her arm in the air and tell her to relax. Then, when I let go of her arm, it stays in the air. . . . or a person who constantly has a sore neck will be on the table, lying on his back, while I try to lift his head. I cannot lift it because the posterior muscles of the neck are rigid. All day, every day, he tightly contracts the muscles in the back of his neck, totally unaware of them, and comes to me wondering why he has constant neck pain.

The answer to the question of why chronic daily headache sufferers are so out of touch with somatic events is extremely complex. As noted previously, their coping strategies of choice—avoiding or ignoring the pain for as long as possible—naturally promote poor awareness. In addition, it might be argued that most people in our culture are out of touch with their own bodies, having learned to rely on external solutions to physical illness, viewing treatment as something that happens to them. Elite athletes certainly cannot be considered representative of the population. Psychobiological aspects of headache are often mistaken by sufferers as being synonymous with a psychological explanation of their condition, leading to the fear that the disorder will be minimized or blamed on them.

There is a suggestion in the literature that headache sufferers, rather than being unaware, are too aware of their headache-related physiology. Pennebaker and Watson (1991) maintain that individuals who complain of a number of psychophysiologic symptoms also exhibit the personality trait of Negative Affectivity (NA), a trait characterized by neuroticism, trait anxiety, and general maladjustment: "High NA individuals appear to be hypervigilant about their bodies and have a lower threshold for noticing and reporting subtle bodily sensations." There is no evidence that chronic daily headache sufferers are prone to amplify body sensations.

Absence of somatic focus may have been adaptive in an evolutionary sense as human functioning would become inefficient if people had to constantly shift attention from external to internal stimuli. The conscious brain may not be designed to simultaneously monitor both internal and external events. Self-defensiveness may also contribute to the lack of somatic awareness. Fisher (1986) maintains that most people do not like to be confronted by their own physical attributes. Most of the literature on this topic deals with external physical attributes or body image. Persons often become uncomfortable when made aware of one or more physical attributes.

Personality and Self-Regulation

There has been, since the early writings of Wolff (1937), an effort to identify personality attributes of headache sufferers in general. There is still no consistent evidence that persons with chronic daily headache, or any particular type of headache, have a single personality style, psychological disorder, or collection of personal attributes. A recent study by Kohler and Kosanic (1992), for example, reexamined the classical question of whether migraineurs are characterized by a high degree of ambition, orderliness and rigidity. They found no differences on these traits between the headache sufferers and matched controls.

When negative traits surrounding anger, anxiety, and depression have been detected in headache sufferers, there remains the issue of whether these factors are best understood as a cause or an effect of headache. There is evidence on both sides of the question. When these variables are considered as traits of the individual, they provide a context in which the headache arises or serves as a marker of a more basic condition that gives rise to both the affective pathology and the headache (Breslau & Davis, 1992).

There is presently some interest in the possibility that chronic daily headache and depression share a unique relationship. Nappi (1991) believes that depression and chronic daily headache may share common biochemical pathways. However, there is presently no compelling evidence that chronic daily headache patients are more depressed prior to headache than are persons in general or headache patients who do not develop daily headache. With pain patients generally, increased pain severity/frequency/duration has been associated with increased depression as measured by questionnaire or structured interview (Haythronthwaite, Sieber, & Kerns, 1991).

The more conservative position is to accept affective pathology in chronic daily headache as a secondary factor that then further aggravates the headache syndrome. This position relies on literature that finds no differences on such variables between headache and nonheadache groups but does find a relationship between pain frequency/severity/duration indices and psychological distress (Cunningham et al., 1987; Andrasik et al., 1988; Blanchard, Kirsch, Appelbaum, & Jaccard 1989; Mongini, Ferla, & Maccagnani, 1991). In this way, the clinician may address the dysphoric affect in treatment as an aggravating factor without having to decide the "chicken and egg" question.

The concept of alexithymia deserves a special mention. It has often been associated with patients who present with chronic physical symptoms not associated with findings of disease. Alexithymia refers to the absence of emotional expressiveness, particularly negative emotions (Taylor, 1984). An example of this cognitive style is contained in the following excerpt from material provided by a patient who was asked to monitor thoughts and feelings that precede changes in pain:

> Saturday: Sore back and head this morning, very foggy out, other than that feel not too bad, very foggy out, rain and snow predicted, when will the sun shine? . . . oat and bran flakes for breakfast with sliced bananas and milk. . . . Later in the day went for a walk with a friend . . . . had difficulty keeping up because of pain. . . . Later in day my sciatic nerve really hurt . . . had difficulty walking because my right side hurt. Walked to grocery store . . . had breast of chicken, tomato and watermelon for dinner . . . pain now worse in head, hands, neck, lower back . . . started new blood pressure medication . . . my

doctor suggested that I may have a rare neurologic disease, something like Parkinson's.

While a number of factors may have been affecting this patient's pain, including weather front, diet, muscle irritation, and secondary neural irritation, the report is notable for the absence of a single reference to emotion. This pattern was repeated over several days until it was discussed and worked with in the course of treatment.

Developing a theoretical/treatment perspective that recognizes the importance of personality but does not demand a one-to-one relationship between personality and headache is crucial. Personality-based reactions appear to affect headache indirectly through a form of collateral psychobiological discharge. Physiologists use the term "collateral" to describe physiological pathways that contribute to nonspecific activation regions such as the somatosensory cortex and noradrenergic pathways. Many factors may affect such activity, including cognitive and somatic activity in response to events that are critical, somatically or psychologically, to the individual. Creditor (1982) stated the situation quite eloquently.

> Although I was frequently unable to attribute a particular attack to a particular circumstance, I was never surprised if an attack was associated with an important event in my life. The emphasis here is on the word "important," because it did not matter whether the event was a happy or a sad one, or whether it had a desirable or an unpleasant outcome. I was never surprised if a migraine occurred *after* a final examination or Board examination, the acceptance of a new position or notification of a promotion, the birth of a child or marriage of a daughter. (p. 1031)

Viewing personality as a corollary construct allows the clinician the flexibility to integrate patients' personal attributes within the context of their psychobiological condition. In this way, it is possible to individualize evaluation and treatment, taking into account the character style of the patient.

The following cases, taken from Sorbi and Tellegen (1988) illustrate how different personality characteristics and coping styles interact with situational factors to influence headache activity:

> Patient no. 10, a married student nurse, displayed a strong positive relation between expression of emotions/anger and

the occurrence of migraine attacks ... attacks typically occurred after being with her parents, whom she visited almost every weekend. Her parents expected her to help a great deal with the cleaning and maintenance of their house. Instead of refusing to cooperate on some of these tasks, she would avoid expressing her irritation and anger and try to meet all of her parents' demands. She would, however, blurt out her negative feelings as soon as she returned to her husband. But at that time a migraine attack would be well on its way.

Patient no. 12, an elderly housewife, presented a strong relation between migraine attacks and comforting cognitions. ... It appeared that attacks occurred often when worrying about her drug-addicted son who was wanted by the police. Although she tried, she was unsuccessful to comfort herself cognitively because of strong interference of anxiety and concern.

Patient no. 16, a socially withdrawn biology student who shared accommodations with other students, showed a marked association between migraine attacks and "social support." ... In her case seeking social support meant lamenting over noise or disturbances from others when in an attack. She otherwise would not share problems with others nor ask for help or advice concerning matters of every-day life. (pp. 355–356).

There is more to headache susceptibility in these individuals than particular occurrences of negative feelings. At the same time, these negative feelings need to be recognized as one of the pieces of the puzzle making up chronic daily headache. We would not necessarily disagree with the psychodynamic position that headache is often maintained by persistent "physiological trouble" resulting from unresolved motives (Adler & Adler, 1987). The goal of understanding, however, remains that of bringing to the patient's awareness the impact of personal motives on headache mechanisms rather than necessarily changing the motives.

Treatment Implications

Chronic daily headache is extremely difficult to change. Biobehavioral interventions involving relaxation training, biofeedback, and cognitive therapy, although routinely utilized in headache clinics, are not as effective with this group as with episodic headache disorders. The treatment failure rate with headaches in general, according to Turk and Rudy (1991), ranges from one-third to one-half. There are data indicating that chronic daily sufferers improve even less. Our early data (Bakal, Demjen, & Kaganov, 1981) showed a reduction of only 11% in posttreatment headache activity (hours per day) following exposure to an intensive biobehavioral treatment program, while subjects in two episodic groups showed an average reduction of 61% and 52%. The cognitive behavioral intervention procedure was clearly not effective for chronic daily headache sufferers.

Blanchard, Appelbaum, Radnitz, Jaccard, and Dentinger (1989), following efforts to treat this population, concluded that daily headache sufferers are refractory to intensive psychological treatment. They compared the effectiveness of a biobehavioral treatment program in reducing headache activity in a group of chronic headache patients who experienced daily headache with two additional groups who experienced either 1–2 headache-free days per week or 3–5 headache-free days per week. The treatment was intensive, involving relaxation training, biofeedback, and cognitive therapy across 8–12 sessions. The episodic headache sufferers showed the usual 50% reduction in headache activity, while the daily headache group showed an improvement of only 13% No explanation was given for the refractory nature of their condition. In a second paper, these investigators (Michulta, Blanchard, Appelbaum, Jaccard, & Dentinger, 1989) reported that daily headache sufferers who did not respond to treatment were also more likely to be using high levels of analgesic medication.

In spite of the difficulties, the approach to chronic daily headache treatment remains that of increasing the use of self-regulation skills in the patient's lifestyle (Duckro, 1991). With this group in particular, it is clear that the use of specific techniques, diets, and medications will not succeed unless the patients learn to better understand the psychobiologic processes that contribute to their daily headache pattern. Interventions have to be highly individualized and reflect the particular patient's characteristics that both enhance and reduce headache susceptibility. Personality and dynamic factors need to be integrated within the self-regulatory skills presented.

The key to self-regulation remains becoming more rather than less aware of body sensations that accompany thoughts, feelings, and behavior. This approach is difficult, since many of these persons lack the proclivity to look inward. It is especially difficult for them to grasp the distinction between preoccupation with their pain and appropriate somatic awareness. Many of these patients also perceive little therapeutic value in the bodily information accessed through somatic awareness. Sometimes it is helpful, in the early stages of treatment, to ask these patients to consider the headache as a chronic disorder over which they cannot have complete control. With this understanding they may be able to set more appropriate goals, looking for management rather than elimination of pain, and appreciating small changes as significant. From these small beginnings they are able to notice early markers of increased severity and moderate less severe pain. With the confidence that some self-regulation is possible, they can proceed to develop hypotheses regarding specific reactions that affect their headache pain and strategies for altering these reactions.

In closing, it is important to emphasize the need for developing better explanatory models for chronic headache sufferers themselves. These individuals have been assured on endless occasions that one form of medication or another will prove effective, only to be disappointed with lack of relief. The treatment paradox facing the medical approach to headache management, regardless of the episodic or daily nature of the condition, is whether, through improved understanding of biochemical mechanisms alone (serotonergic system, 5 HT receptors, trigeminovascular system, and neurogenic inflammation) we are ensuring that headache sufferers remain convinced that they have little or no role to play in the treatment process. Efforts to explain the disorder at purely psychological levels fare no better. It is vital that these patients understand that using biobehavioral techniques does not imply that their headache is a "psych problem."

Adoption by patients of a self-regulatory philosophy will be greatly enhanced with improved understanding of the meaning and nature of the psychobiologic determinants of their condition. As long as headache remains a mysterious and poorly understood phenomenon, we can expect these individuals to continue to adopt coping strategies that are maladaptive and ineffective (Williams & Keefe, 1991). They must understand that while headache is an inherited propensity with a definite neurophysiological substrate, it is also a condition that is inextricably tied to their thoughts, feelings, and bodily sensations. Regulating the complex processes involved is best achieved by developing enduring and overriding habits of somatic awareness.

References

Adler, C. S., & Adler, S. M. (1987). Psychodynamics of head pain: An introduction. In C. S. Adler, S. M. Adler, & R. C. Packard (Eds.), *Psychiatric aspects of headache* (pp. 41–55). Baltimore: Williams & Wilkins.

Amery, W. K., Waelkens, J., & Vandenbergh, V. (1986). Migraine warnings. *Headache, 26,* 60–66.

Andrasik, F., Kabela, E., Quinn, S., Attanasio, V., Blanchard, E. B., & Rosenblum, E. L. (1988). Psychological functioning of children who have recurrent migraine. *Pain, 34,* 43–52.

Bakal, D. A. (1982). *Psychobiology of chronic headache.* New York: Springer Publishing Co.

Bakal, D. A., Demjen, S., & Kaganov, J. (1984). The continuous nature of headache susceptibility. *Social Science & Medicine, 19,* 1305–1311.

Blanchard, E. B., Appelbaum, K. A., Radnitz, C. L., Jaccard, J., & Dentinger, M. P. (1989). The refractory headache patient—I. Two studies of Chronic, Daily, High Intensity Headache. *Behaviour Research and Therapy, 27,* 403–410.

Blanchard, E. B., Kirsch, C. A., Appelbaum, K. A., & Jaccard, J. (1989). Role of psychopathology in chronic headache: Cause or effect. *Headache, 29,* 295–301.

Breslau, N., & Davis, G. C. (1992). Migraine, major depression and panic disorder: A prospective epidemiologic study of adults. *Cephalgia, 12,* 85–90.

Cantwell-Simmons, E., Duckro, P. N., & Richardson, W. D. (1993). A review of studies on the relationship of chronic analgesic use and chronic headache. *Headache Quarterly: Current Treatment and Research, 4,* 28–35.

Cioffi, D. (1991). Beyond attentional strategies: A cognitive-perceptual model of somatic interpretation. *Psychological Bulletin, 109,* 25–41.

Creditor, M. C. (1982). Me and migraine. *The New England Journal of Medicine, 307,* 1029–1032.

Cunningham, S. J., McGrath, P. J., Ferguson, H. B., Humphreys, P., D'Astous, J., Latter, J., Goodman, J. T., & Firestone, P. (1987). Personality and behavioural characteristics in pediatric migraine. *Headache, 27,* 16–20.

Demjen, S., Bakal, D. A., & Dunn, B. E. (1990). Cognitive correlates of headache intensity and duration. *Headache, 30,* 423–427.

Dexter, J. D. (1987). The relationship between headache syndromes and sleep. In C. S. Adler, S. M. Adler, & R. C. Packard (Eds.), *Psychiatric aspects of headache* (pp. 254–258). Baltimore: Williams & Wilkins.

Diener, H. C., Dichgans, J., Scholz, E., Geiselhart, S., Gerber, W. D., & Bille, A. (1989). Analgesic-induced chronic headache: Long-term results of withdrawal therapy. *Journal of Neurology, 236,* 9–14.

Duckro, P. N. (1990). Biofeedback in the management of headache: Part I. *Headache Quarterly, 1,* 290–298.

Duckro, P. N. (1991). Biofeedback in the management of headache: Part II. *Headache Quarterly, 2,* 17–22.

Fisher, S. (1986). *Development and structure of the body image (vol. 1).* Hillsdale, NJ: Lawrence Erlbaum Associates.

Hanna, T. (1988). *Somatics.* Reading, MA: Addison-Wesley.

Hatch, J.P., Prihoda, T.J., Moore, P.J., Cyr-Provost, M., Borcherding, S., Boutros, N.N., & Seleshi, E. (1991). A naturalistic study of the relationships among electromyographic activity, psychological stress, and pain in ambulatory tension-type headache patients and headache-free controls. *Psychosomatic Medicine, 53,* 576–584.

Haythornthwaite, J.A., Sieber, W.J., & Kerns, R.D. (1991). Depression and the chronic pain experience. *Pain, 46,* 177–184.

Headache Classification Committee of the International Headache Society. (1988). Classification and diagnostic criteria for headache disorders, cranial neuralgias and facial pain. *Cephalgia, 8, Supplement 7.*

Kohler, T., & Kosanic, S. (1992). Are persons with migraine characterized by a high degree of ambition, orderliness, and rigidity? *Pain, 48,* 321–323.

Mathew, N. T. (1991). Chronic daily headache: Clinical features and natural history. In G. Nappi, G. Bono, G. Sandrini, E. Martignomi, & G. Micieli (Eds.), *Headache and depression: Serotonin pathways as a common cause* (pp. 49–58). New York: Raven.

McCaul, K. D., & Malott, J. M. (1984). Distraction and coping with pain. *Psychological Bulletin, 95,* 516–533.

Michulta, D. M., Blanchard, E. B., Appelbaum, K. A., Jaccard, J., & Dentinger, M. P. (1989). The refractory headache patient—II. High medication consumption (analgesic rebound) headache. *Behaviour Research and Therapy, 27,* 411–420.

Moldofsky, H. (1989). Sleep and Fibrositis Syndrome. *Rheumatic Disease Clinics, 15,* 91–103.

Mongini, F., Ferla, E., & Maccagnani, C. (1991). MMPI profiles in patients with headache or craniofacial pain: A comparative study. *Cephalgia, 12,* 91–98.

Morgan, W., & Pollock, M. (1977). Psychologic characterization of the elite distance runner. *Annals of the New York Academy of Sciences, 301,* 382–403.

Nappi, G. (1991). Introduction: Headache and depression. In G. Nappi, G. Bono, G. Sandrini, E. Martignomi, & G. Micieli (Eds.), *Headache and depression: Serotonin pathways as a common clue* (pp. ix–xi). New York, Raven.

Olesen, J. (1991). Clinical and pathophysiological observations in migraine and tension-type headache explained by integration of vascular, supraspinal and myofascial inputs. *Pain, 46,* 125–132.

Ostfeld, A. M., & Wolff, H. H. (1958). Identification, mechanisms and management of the migraine syndrome. *Medical Clinics of North America, 42,* 1497–1509.

Pennebaker, J. W., & Watson, D. (1991). The psychology of somatic symptoms. In L. J. Kirmayer & J. M. Robbins (Eds.), *Current concepts of somatization: Research and clinical perspectives.* Washington, DC: American Psychiatric Press.

Philips, H. C. (1987). Avoidance behaviour and its role in sustaining chronic pain. *Behaviour Research and Therapy, 25,* 273–279.

Rosenstiel, A. K., & Keefe, F. J. (1983). The use of coping strategies in chronic low back pain patients: Relationship to patient characteristics and current adjustment. *Pain, 17,* 33–40.

Saper, J. (1988). Daily chronic headache—Tension headaches, migraine, and combined headaches: The transformational concept. In H. C. Diener & M. Wilkinson (Eds.), *Drug-induced headache* (pp. 5–7). New York: Springer-Verlag.

Saper, J. R., Johnson, T., & van Meter, M. (1983). "Mixed headache." A chronic headache complex: A study of 500 patients (Abstract). *Headache, 23,* 143.

Schoenen, J., Gerard, P., De Pasqua, V., & Juprelle, M. (1991). EMG activity in pericranial muscles during postural variation and mental activity in healthy volunteers and patients with chronic tension type headache. *Headache, 31,* 321–324.

Sorbi, M., & Tellegen, B. (1988). Stress-coping in migraine. *Social Science & Medicine, 26,* 351–358.

Spinhoven, P., Jochems, P. A., Linssen, A. C. G., & Bogaards, M. (1991). The relationship of personality variables and patient recruitment to pain coping strategies and psychological distress in tension headache patients. *The Clinical Journal of Pain, 7,* 12–20.

Taylor, G. J. (1984). Alexithymia: Concept, measurement, and implications for treatment. *American Journal of Psychiatry, 141,* 725–732.

Turk, D. C., & Rudy, T. E. (1991). Neglected topics in the treatment of chronic pain patients—relapse, noncompliance, and adherance enhancement. *Pain, 44,* 5–28.

Tyrer, P., Casey, P., & Ferguson, B. (1991). Personality disorder in perspective. *British Journal of Psychiatry, 159,* 463–471.

Walls, E. W., & Philipp, E. E. (1953). *Hilton's rest and pain* (6th ed.). London: G. Bell & Sons. (First published in 1863 by Bell and Daldy, London).

Wilkinson, M. (1988). Introduction. In H. C. Diener & M. Wilkinson (Eds.), *Drug-induced headache* (pp. 1–2). New York: Springer-Verlag.

Williams, D. A., & Keefe, F. J. (1991). Pain beliefs and the use of cognitive-behavioral coping strategies. *Pain, 46,* 185–190.

Wolff, H. G. (1937). Personality features and reactions of subjects with migraine. *Archives of Neurology and Psychiatry, 37,* 895–921.

Chapter Six

Attachment and Pain

David J. Anderson and Robert H. Hines

Pain is an amazingly complex and mysterious phenomenon. It is not merely a sensation, but an experience that provokes the imagination, memory, and emotions of the afflicted and challenges the patient and physician to comprehend it. The person with pain seeks the help of the caregiver (often a physician) to bring this noxious experience to an end. It is in and through the relationship with the caregiver that the pain experience may be resolved. Most physicians relate to their patients through the prescription of medication, exercise, and procedures (diagnostic and therapeutic). The manner in which the patient consciously and unconsciously interprets these interventions may be critical in determining the outcome of the pain experience.

Early in our work with patients with chronic refractory spine pain, we observed that patients with certain childhood experiences that were potentially damaging to the development of healthy secure attachment were much more likely to fail after surgery and/or conservative care. The converse also appeared to be true. What we will present in this chapter is a model that places the patient's attachment history at the center of our thinking about the pain experience and the vulnerability to pain. We hypothesize that an individual's capacity to be consoled (i.e., recover from the pain inducing injury) is directly related to his or her attachment security. The more insecure the attachment, the less consolable the person will be and, as a result, the more vulnerable to chronic pain. Thus, the inability to tolerate and accommodate to pain can be predicted by the lack of a secure base in childhood with its resultant insecure attachment. Conversely, the presence of such a secure base and the resulting secure attachment is correlated with an ability to tolerate and accommodate to pain.

In 1982 we were asked to join a team of physicians who were evaluating and treating people with spine pain of various etiologies. The principal phenomenon that we were asked to investigate was the observation that some patients with objective structural pathology were not recovering as expected despite technically good surgical outcomes. Although some of these failures were explained by the physicians as being due to the patients' being "hysterical," many of the patients were viewed as "solid citizens" whose failure perplexed the physicians and led to extraordinary diagnostic investigations and further unsuccessful surgery. Our task was to discover the psychological and psychosocial factors that might be contributing to these patients' failure to recover and to develop effective treatment to avert or reverse failure.

Previous psychological and psychiatric input had relied on the Minnesota Multiphasic Personality Inventory (MMPI) and the Millon Behavioral Health Inventory, as well as cognitive and behavioral assessment of the patients. In our experience these evaluations only gave the team a diagnostic label or a description of the patient's character style under stress. Unfortunately, this information usually only confirmed the impressions of the primary physicians that the patient was "hysterical" or a "psych case" and did not suggest a plan for treatment that could be integrated into the medical care.

Over the last 10 years, we have evaluated nearly 5,000 patients. Nearly two-thirds of these patients have been followed prospectively, ranging from a single follow-up visit to weekly psychotherapy lasting 4 years. Though our model has grown out of our clinical work with patients having spine pain, we suggest that it is applicable to other painful medical conditions as well.

Working with patients having disabling spine pain has taught us a great deal about the nature of the spine pain experience and its resolution. By studying the processes of adjustment, assimilation, and adaptation that patients utilize to recover from a spine injury we have been able to discern a recurrent pattern of affective and cognitive challenges that confront the individual with spine pain (Anderson & Moskowitz, 1991). These challenges exist to a varying degree for every patient and are an outcome of the unique and vital functions that the spine performs for everyone. If these functions were not central to human existence, we believe that the problem of disabling spine pain would be much less significant. This recovery process encompasses an inexorable loss of the patient's former identity and way of life. The discovery and implementation of a new way of being and doing that incorporates the injured spine must follow. Though highly variable in intensity and degree of disruption, the psychological challenges inherent in the recovery process spare no one. If a patient circumvents the process and attempts to return without changes to his former life, the recovery will be short lived, and often the pain will return with greater intensity.

To more fully appreciate the challenges of the recovery process, the particular meanings of the lumbar spine to the human psyche must be appreciated. Fundamentally, it is the lumbar spine that provides the base of support for the human species' upright posture, which in part makes our species unique. It is this very upright posture and all the autonomous acitivity it allows that is put in jeopardy by the back injury.

Unremitting back pain threatens to evoke a level of dependency that few individuals have experienced since before they first stood. With the onset of locomotion, the 1-year-old child assumes an upright posture. This developmental period is marked by a seeming increase in independence and autonomy. Mahler described this phase of a child's development as the "practicing subphase of separation-individuation" (Mahler, Pine, & Bergman, 1975). During this developmental period the child uses the security of his relationship with his mother to more actively and enthusiastically explore the world. Indeed, the world is much more within the toddler's grasp. While the 1-year-old is able to seek out and explore with seeming impunity, it is always within the security net of a watchful caregiver and only with frequent check-ins for "emotional refueling" (Mahler et al., 1975).

Importantly, the preupright period is also without expressive language, just as in many ways the spine pain experience is beyond words. The lack of the ability for verbal communication of the experience makes it extremely difficult to relate to the caregiver. Even those words that are available in everyday metaphoric language are rather disparaging. If someone is accused of being "spineless," it is to suggest a cowardly avoidance of responsibility. People are urged to have "more backbone" when being admonished to be more decisive and more independent. We "break our backs" when we work diligently under burdensome circumstances, especially when it involves a martyred sense of duty. We "bend over backwards" when inordinate and flexible generosity is required by another's insistent demands. Thus when stricken by back pain, an ominous threat of potentially humiliating and indescribable dependency that does not allow us to stand up for ourselves (have backbone), work hard (break our backs), or have any flexibility in the face of everyday demands (bend over backwards) ensues. It is apparent from this "body" language that the spine allows the human being far more than just upright posture.

The model that we will present is further rooted in observations first made by researchers in two independent fields over 30 years ago. George Engel, in his insightful paper entitled "Psychogenic Pain and the Pain-Prone Patient" (1959), hypothesized that various constellations of childhood psychological neglect and abuse established a proclivity towards the development of pain in excess to what would be expected for the known peripheral pain generator. He based his hypothesis on repeated histories of such abuse in patients with chronic pain. His explanations were limited to psychoanalytical speculations that did not make practical intervention accessible. As a result, his observations have not received much corroborative attention except for a recent study by Adler et al., who found support for Engel's impressions in a controlled retrospective study (Adler, Zlot, Hurny, & Minder, 1989).

While Engel was working with patients having chronic pain, other researchers in child development were empirically studying the natural development of attachment in early human relationships between children and significant caregivers (e.g., Bowlby, 1958; Ainsworth, Bell, & Slayton, 1971). What they observed and described provides a sound theoretical framework for Engel's observations.

John Bowlby, drawing considerable inspiration from ethology and the previous observations of Konrad Lorenz on imprinting in birds, turned the psychoanalytic world on its ear by introducing his theory of attachment. Despite the observations of Spitz (1945) on the devastating consequences of early maternal deprivation, psychoanalytic theory prior to Bowlby generally considered feeding as the primary force in the maternal tie with an infant, resulting in dependency. Bowlby, in the 1950s and 1960s, laid the groundwork for the primacy of an internally driven pattern of behaviors that lead to attachment (1958, 1982). Bowlby conceptualized attachment as a fundamental form of behavior no less important in motivation than feeding or sex and no less important for survival. Attachment has a protective function in assuring proximity of a primary caregiver during times of great vulnerability in childhood. Attachment behaviors are also evident during times of stress or sickness. It is our observation that they are also evoked by spine injury and its resultant pain.

Mary Salter Ainsworth, who had studied with Bowlby and others at the Tavistock Clinic, led the field with a flood of empirical studies that validated and augmented the clinical significance of attachment theory. In her now seminal work, using Harlow's (1961) work with rhesus monkeys as inspiration, she designed a study observing separation and reunion of 1-year-olds with their mothers in a strange situation (Ainsworth & Wittig, 1969). She was struck by the infants' behavior on reunion and the similarity to observations made earlier at Tavistock while she was with Bowlby and others. Three main groups of infants were identified on the basis of their behavior in the strange situation. The preponderance of infants fell into a group that showed active play and exploration in the mother's presence, enthusiastic greetings of mother upon her return from separation, seeking of contact with mother upon her return with consolation as a result, and contact-seeking by both mother and infant despite any apparent negative feedback. The other groups, which in the original study were identified as *anxiously attached*, have received more descriptive labels over time (Ainsworth, Blehar, Water, & Wall, 1978). One group of the anxiously attached was seen as "insecure–avoidant" and the other as "insecure–ambivalent." The insecure–avoidant children did not use their mother as a base of reassurance and seemed oblivious to her comings and goings. The insecure–ambivalent children showed distress on their mother's leaving and were inconsolable even when mother returned.

Stroufe, among others, has shown that individual differences in quality of attachment are related to quality of caregiving (1983). Other longitudinal studies have demonstrated the cross-cultural applicability of maternal sensitivity and quality of attachment

(Grossman, Grossman, & Spangler, 1985). Avoidant attachments are correlated to hostile aversion, or "emotional unavailability" (Stroufe, 1983). Consistently abused children are highly likely to show avoidant attachments. Ambivalent attachments are correlated with inconsistent nurturing without active aversion such as might be seen with inadequate care or simple physical neglect. More recently, Main (1991), upon review of videotapes of strange situation behaviors of infants not heretofore classified, found yet another class of insecurely attached infants who demonstrated "disorganized or disoriented behaviors." While specific parental behaviors associated with this type of insecure attachment are not known, unresolved trauma (e.g., loss of a parent or sexual abuse) is postulated.

The predictive value of types of attachments for future development is now well ensconced in the developmental literature. "The weight of evidence would seem to support the belief that the emotional system of childhood attachment is the parent system for the emotional systems of adult attachment" (Weiss, 1991). Indeed, longitudinal studies have shown or are showing that attachment patterns are stable across one's life span (Grossman & Grossman, 1991; Main, 1988). Not only do the types of communication between the infant and caregiver persist but other developmental outcomes are evident. Securely attached infants tend to make a successful adjustment to preschool, whereas an anxious attachment is a strong predictor of kindergarten retention. Emotional independence, high self-esteem, and empathy for and competence with peers are also predicted by secure attachment. Avoidant attachments are predictive of hostile aggression towards other children and alienation of teachers as well as being strongly associated with childhood depression. Ambivalent attachments are generally predictive of immaturity and impulsivity (Stroufe, 1985). The stability of patterns of attachment has been repeatedly established (Egeland, Byron, & Stroufe, 1981; Stroufe, 1983; Grossman & Grossman, 1991; Weiss, 1991). Bowlby suggested as an explanation for the stability of these patterns that "expectancies and self-fulfilling prophecies increase the stability of internal models" (Grossman & Grossman, 1991). While changing life events, support from family, or other positive influences on caregiver sensitivity may modify the type of attachment (Egeland, Byron, & Stroufe, 1981), the absence of a secure base in early childhood clearly has devastating and permanent consequences. Given the repeating pattern of child–caregiver interactions suggested by Bowlby (1982), a template of expectations, behavior, and even neurophysiological responses develop in the individual. At times of stress such as loss, illness, or certainly (in our experience) with back injury, attachment behavior is increased, and, when it is based on lack of a secure base, it becomes maladaptive.

As yet, no objective scale of attachment has been developed. As a result, indirect measures must be used that either reflect the quality of attachments or factors known to disrupt attachment. Initially, we designed a 100-item questionnaire to evaluate the extent of disturbing factors in the patient's attachment history. When this questionnaire proved to be cumbersome, we consolidated and simplified the factors potentially damaging to the development of a secure attachment to five types of experiences. These factors are by no means complete, and patients without any of these risk factors may have insecure attachments and be missed by these criteria. Nevertheless, these factors provide a gross indirect predictor of quality of attachment. Each factor was assessed during the course of a semi-structured clinical interview based on the Adult Attachment Interview (George, Kaplan, & Main, 1984; Main, 1991).

These childhood experiences are considered factors that, if present, could endanger the establishment of a secure attachment and lead to increased vulnerability to pain. For our model, we define childhood as the period before the age of 21, and a primary caregiver as a parent or other significant adult entrusted to care for the child. While very early experiences are perhaps most relevant to security of attachment, attachment patterns tend to persist and be repeated throughout life. The factors are:

1. *Physical abuse*: present if the patient suffered a physical injury inflicted by the primary caregiver that was not accidental. The effects of physical abuse on attachment have been well established. Recent studies with abused and neglected children using the "strange situation" paradigm confirm the grave consequences of violence in the family on security of attachment (Crittenden, 1992).
2. *Sexual Abuse*: present if a primary caregiver or other adult abused or exploited the child for the caregiver's sexual stimulation. The role of sexual abuse in the development of inse-

cure attachments has been recently reviewed (Alexander, 1992).

3. *Alcohol or Drug Abuse in One or Both of the Primary Caregivers*: present if the patient states that the caregiver had problems with the use of alcohol or drugs. Not only does drug use in pregnancy affect the unborn child's security of attachment, but substance-abusing mothers score negatively on variables of attachment more frequently than nonusing mothers (Wachsman, Schuetz, & Chan, 1989).

4. *Abandonment*: present if the patient suffered the loss of a primary caregiver that the patient perceived as abandonment. The adverse effects of repeated threats to abandon, let alone abandonment itself, on security of attachment was discussed by Bowlby (1988) in his book, *A Secure Base*.

5. *Emotional Neglect/Abuse*: present if the patient relates that the primary caregiver(s) were not available for emotional support or were actively and persistently critical, demanding, or rejecting of the child's emotional needs. Some of the most compelling evidence for the untoward effect of emotional unavailability on security attachment comes from studies of children of depressed caregivers (Radke-Yarrow, 1991).

In our retrospective study we were able to confirm a relationship between childhood psychological trauma and poor surgical outcome (Schofferman, Anderson, Hines, Smith, & White, 1992). A clear and significant correlation was demonstrated between the number of childhood risk factors (roughly equivalent to the severity of damage to attachment security) and the success rate of lumbar spine surgery. Patients who have had three or more risk factors had an 85% failure rate, whereas those with none had only a 5% failure rate. Conversely, in patients with a poor surgical outcome, the prevalence of three or more risk factors was 75 percent. The correlation was seen in single-level, multi-level, primary, and repeat surgeries and increased progressively and with statistical significance with each additional risk factor. Factor analysis was not done to determine the relative strength of each risk factor or which combination of risk factors might be more damaging to attachment security.

It is important to emphasize that it is not necessarily the presence of abuse or neglect in the history of the patient, but the effects such events may have had on the capacity of the individual to form consoling relationships (i.e., secure attachments). Some patients have a significant history of neglect or abuse but have found sanctuary through their relationship with a nurturing adult such as a high school coach, a favorite teacher, or a relative. Others less fortunate have found refuge not in human relationships but in physical activities such as athletics and physical work. Such consoling havens are severely disrupted by spine pain, leaving the individual without his familiar consoling activity.

Central to our understanding of vulnerability to pain is the adverse effect on security of attachment that childhood traumas play. It is the presence of such traumas, particularly when repetitive, that is disturbing and potentially damaging to attachment security. In addition, it is from the secure base that attachment can provide that one not only explores the world, but also weathers the inevitable traumas of life. Several investigators have found a high incidence of early adverse childhood experiences in adults with painful medical illnesses (Wurtele, Kaplan, Keairnes, 1990; Domino, & Haber, 1987; Walker, et al., 1988). The focus in these studies was on the experiences alone and not on the effects that the experiences had on attachment. To better understand how these early childhood experiences damage attachment, it is necessary to provide at least an introduction to the psychology, neuropsychology, and neurophysiology of trauma.

Van der Kolk, a prominent psychiatric researcher in psychological trauma, states that traumatization occurs when both internal and external resources are "inadequate to cope with an external threat to one's existence" (1989, p. 404). Trauma leads to hyperarousal states for which the victim's memory of the event can be state dependent or entirely dissociated. This hyperarousal state persists as chronic to the extent that the trauma is not adequately resolved and integrated (van der Kolk, 1989). Thus a trauma only threatens to disturb the underlying attachment but if the caregiver's interventions are inadequate, then the consequences of the trauma may persist. That is, lack of adequate consolation by the caregiver or lack of receptivity to such consolation serves to perpetuate the sequelae of the trauma such as in hyperarousal. Physiologic hyperarousal is activated by stimuli reminiscent of the trauma. These stresses or stimuli tend to be experienced as nonspecific somatic states (e.g., tics, tremors, wheezing, pain, panic attacks) rather than as new specific events that require specific means of coping. Van der Kolk (1989) states that:

> Trauma victims may respond to contemporary stimuli as if a return of the trauma has occurred without the conscious awareness that it is a *past* [italics added] injury (e.g., physical or sexual abuse, abandonment) and *not* [italics added] the current conscious stress that is identified by them that is responsible for the emergency hyperarousal state. (p. 405)

Trauma also induces long-term potentiation of memory tracts (flashbacks) that are also reactivated at times of subsequent arousal. Cognitively, this hyperarousal interferes with the victim's ability to make rational assessments of his experience and prevents resolution and integration of the previous trauma and the current stresses. In addition, disturbances in the brain's catecholamines, serotonin, and endorphins participate in this confusing hyperaroused state. Further understanding of these biochemical disturbances is important if pharmacological interventions are to become effective in facilitating resolution of the trauma.

As early attachment patterns are being established, unmitigated trauma serve to disrupt their security. Traumata themselves only threaten the underlying attachment. It is the response of the caregiver to such traumas that is critical. If the caregiver's interventions are inadequate, absent, or additionally traumatic, the trauma becomes enduring and threatens the security of attachment. With anxious attachments also comes a hyperarousal pattern that can be incited by various stresses or stimuli without any conscious link to earlier trauma. This hyperarousal pattern becomes a part of the insecure attachment template. Van der Kolk's work on the effects of trauma supports this interdependent relationship between attachment, vulnerability to trauma, and trauma (van der Kolk, Perry, & Herman, 1991). He suggests that "vulnerability to posttraumatic stress disorder can be predicted on the *security of attachment* and that uncontrollable disruptions or distortions of attachment bonds precede the development of posttraumatic stress syndromes" (van der Kolk, 1989). Clearly, trauma and attachment are interdependent phenomena. Underlying any disturbed attachment are the latent hyperarousal, biochemical, and cognitive states of the earlier causative trauma. These states await reactivation by any stress that threatens links to current attachment figures.

BRAIN
(to areas that underlie pain experience & localization)

Tonic influences from
Cortex and Midbrain
(Cultural, personality,
factors)

Intermittent brain influences
(attention, anxiety, and
hyperarousal states)

Central Pain

Generating

Descending inhibitions
from the Brainstem

Visceral Inputs
(e.g., nausea)

Chronic neural changes
from prolonged
noxious stimulation

Mechanism

Autonomic Nervous System
inputs

Tonic sensory inputs
(trigger points; scar tissue)

Phasic Sensory Input
(injury and other brief
stimulation)

FIGURE 6.1 Central pattern-generating mechanism to explain various pain phenomena.

Just as unresolved trauma establishes a self-perpetuating chronic hyperarousal pattern, so too can unresolved pain. Over the years, Melzack and his associates have led the way in modern pain research by making fundamental contributions to our understanding of pain (Melzack & Wall, 1982). Both Livingston (1943) and Melzack (1986) suggest that prolonged intense pain or even low-level pain produces self-sustaining neural activity that creates memory-like processes related to chronic pain. Melzack expands this notion in his proposal of a central pattern-generating mechanism (Figure 6.1) to explain various pain phenomena, including chronic pain (Melzack & Loeser, 1978). This mechanism creates the final sensory input to the parts of the brain that underlie the pain experience and localization of pain. This neural pattern is the product of multiple and complex inputs and interactions at all levels of the spinal cord and brain. Melzack (1986) said that inputs include tonic and phasic ones from the brain, such as *"cultural, personality, past experience, expectations, attentional and anxiety variables"* (p. 1). He states "there is no denying the role of neuromas, nerve injury, herniated discs, and so forth as major contributions to pain

. . . but once the abnormal central pattern generating processes are underway the peripheral contributions may assume less importance. . . . Once the pattern generating mechanisms become capable of producing patterns for pain, *any* input may act as a trigger" (Melzack, 1986, p. 29).

Though inclusive of a greater variety of sensory input than van der Kolk's model of unresolved trauma, Melzack's model of the mechanism underlying chronic pain places central modulating influences as a major contributor, and often the sustaining contributor, to pain (Melzack, 1986). These central influences, in our estimation, are most influenced by the attachment/trauma experience of the individual. The more secure the attachment (adequate consolation with early traumas), the more inhibiting of pain is the central influence. The more insecure the attachment (inadequate consolation and hyperarousal), the more facilitating of pain this central influence becomes.

We suggest that as a result of hundreds of interactions between child and caregivers throughout childhood, a unique template of expectations, neurophysiological responses, and behavior develops within the individual that correlate with attachment behavior. This template becomes activated when physical and/or emotional stress is sufficient to threaten one's security. Spine pain and the actual, for some traumatic, ordeal of surgery does activate such templates and expose the weakness or vulnerability of the individual. Once activated, much of the neurophysiology underlying the maintenance of chronic pain becomes operational through the system so eloquently described by van der Kolk (1989) and Melzack (1986).

The findings from research on attachment, as well as our increasing evidence for the long-term effects of disturbances of attachment on pain, present the need for further research on the sequelae of childhood antecedents as well as assessment of therapeutic interventions. Neurophysiological and neuroendocrinological correlates to types of attachment need to be elucidated. Grossman and Grossman (1991) suggest that the factors that may influence changes toward a more secure attachment in adults include psychotherapy, supportive spouses, and emotionally significant others. Valliant (1977), in a prospective study of 100 male Harvard graduates, similarly found that the presence of long-term sustaining relationships in adults was not only positively correlated with emotional and physical health but was a means of overcoming the untoward effects of unhappy childhoods. Certainly, these observations are consonant with our clinical experience: where evidence for insecure attachment exists, strategic interventions are imperative. For those patients who are not responding as expected to conservative care or are being evaluated for possible surgery, treatment planning begins with identification of factors from a developmental history that may make overcoming the rigors of a major surgery or rehabilitation problematic. When identified, surgical intervention should be considered cautiously and only with adequate strategic psychological intervention. Such intervention is necessary not only to enhance the outcome of surgical and/or conservative care but also to avoid simply evoking and not treating previous unresolved traumas and adding further to the patient's inconsolability.

Kolb (1982) has proposed an attachment theory based model of managing chronic-pain patients. Though his model does not include the vulnerability aspects of our model, he does agree "that establishment of a trusting, expectant, and secure attachment base forms the fulcrum on which rests application of any indicated technical intervention to relieve painful distress" (1982, p. 416). It is our experience that the ability of the treatment team to form a consoling relationship with the patient is necessary for a successful outcome. This relationship sometimes entails a psychotherapeutic relationship in the more traditional sense in which the "pain" of an upbringing in which caregivers abrogated their responsibility can be safely explored. Other times it involves the patient successfully finding solace in the group environment such as the variety of 12-step survivor groups or chronic pain groups. At still other times it may involve helping to find the appropriate (e.g., gender, character style, etc.) physical therapist or clinician with whom the patient can relate and form a consoling relationship. The mental health professional in these situations must often serve as the consultant to the other professionals, as the template of insecure attachments usually serves to provoke significant negative responses in other caregivers that can easily serve to perpetuate the patient's internal expectation of traumatizing relationships. In the model we have proposed, chronic pain often represents a nonspecific plea for help in overcoming earlier unresolved traumas, traumas that have disrupted the most basic of human needs—a secure attachment.

References

Adler, R. H., Zlot, S., Hurny, C. & Minder, C. (1989). Psychogenic pain and the pain-prone patient: A retrospective, controlled clinical study. *Psychosomatic medicine, 51*, 87–101.

Ainsworth, M. D. S., & Wittig, B. A. (1969). Attachment and the exploratory behavior of 1-year olds in a strange situation. In B. M. Foss (Ed.), *Determinants of infant behavior, Vol. 4* (pp. 113–136). London: Methuen.

Ainsworth, M. D. S., Bell, S. M. V., & Slayton, D. (1971). Individual differences in strange situation behavior in one-year olds. In H. R. Schaffer (Ed.), *The origins of human social relations.* London: Academic.

Ainsworth, M. D. S., Blehar, M., Water, E., & Wall, S. (1978). *Patterns of attachment: A psychological study of the strange situation.* New York: Basic Books.

Alexander, P. C. (1992). Application of attachment theory to the study of sexual abuse. *Journal of Consulting and Clinical Psychology, 60*(2), 185–195.

Anderson, D. J., & Moskowitz, M. H. (1991). Psychiatric aspects of spine pain. In A. H. White & R. Anderson (Eds.), *Conservative care of back pain* (pp. 274–288). Baltimore: Williams & Wilkins.

Bowlby, J. (1958). The nature of the child's tie to his mother. *International Journal of Psycho-Analysis, 42*, 317–340.

Bowlby, J. (1982). *Attachment*, Vol. 1 of *Attachment and loss* (2nd ed.). New York: Basic Books.

Bowlby, J. (1988). *A secure base.* New York: Basic Books.

Crittenden, P. M. (1992). Childrens' strategies for coping with adverse home environments: An interpretation using attachment theory. *Child Abuse and Neglect, 16*(3), 329–343.

DeLozier, P. (1982). Attachment theory and child abuse. In C. M. Parkes & J. Stevenson-Hinde (eds.), *The place of attachment in human behavior* (pp. 95–117). New York: Basic Books.

Domino, J., & Haber, J. (1987). Prior physical and sexual abuse in women with chronic headache. *Headache, 27*, 310–314.

Egeland, B., Byron, P. & Stroufe, L. A. (1981). Attachment and early maltreatment. *Child Development, 52*, 44–52.

Engel, G. L. (1959). "Psychogenic" pain and the pain-prone patient. *American Journal of Medicine, 26*, 899–918.

George, C., Kaplan, N., & Main, M. (1984). *Attachment interview for adults.* University of California, Berkeley (unpublished manuscript).

Grossman, K., & Grossman, K. E. (1991). Attachment quality as an organizer of emotional and behavioral responses in a longitudinal perspective. In C. M. Parkes, J. Stevenson Hinde, & P. Morris (Eds.), *Attachment across the life cycle* (pp. 93–114). London: Tavistock/Rutledge.

Grossman, K., Grossman, K. E., & Spangler, G. (1985). Maternal sensitivity and newborns' responses as related to quality of attachment in Northern

Germany. In I. Bretherton & E. Waters (eds.), Growing points of attachment theory and research (*Monographs of the Society for Research in Child Development, 50*, Serial No. 209, 1–2).

Harlow, H. F. (1961). The development of affectional patterns in infant monkeys. In B. M. Foss (Ed.), *Determinants of infant behavior* (pp. 75–97). New York: Wiley.

Kolb, L. (1982). Attachment behaviors and pain complaints. *Psychosomatics, 23*, 4, 413–425.

Livingston, W. K. (1943). *Pain mechanisms.* New York: Macmillan.

Mahler, M. S., Pine, F., & Bergman, A. (1975). *The psychological birth of the human infant.* New York: Basic Books.

Main, M. (1991). Metacognitive knowledge, metacognitive monitoring, and singular (coherent) versus multiple (incoherent) models of attachment. In C. M. Parkes, J. Stevenson-Hinde, & P. Morris (Eds.), *Attachment across the life cycle* (pp. 127–159). London: Tavistock/Rutledge.

Main, M., & Cassidy, J. (1988). Categories of response to reunion with the parent at age 6: Predictable from infant attachment classifications and stable over a one month period. *Developmental Psychology, 24*(3), 415–426.

Melzack, R. (1986). Neurophysiological foundations of pain. In R. A. Sternbach (Ed.), *The psychology of pain.* New York: Raven.

Melzack, R., & Loeser, J. D. (1978). Phantom body pain in paraplegics: Evidence for a central "pattern generating mechanism" for pain. *Pain, 4*, 195–210.

Melzack, R., & Wall, P. D. (1982). *The challenge of pain.* New York: Basic Books.

Radke-Yarrow, M. (1991). Attachment patterns in children of depressed mothers. In C. M. Parkes, J. Stevenson-Hinde, & P. Morris (Eds.), *Attachment across the life cycle* (pp. 115–127). London: Tavistock/Rutledge.

Schofferman, J., Anderson, D., Hines, R., Smith, G., & White, A. (1992). Childhood psychological trauma correlates with unsuccessful lumbar spine surgery. *Spine, 17* (Suppl), S138–144.

Stroufe, L. A. (1983). Infant-caregiver attachment and patterns of adaptatiion in pre-school. The roots of maladaptation and competence. In L. H. Perlmutter (Ed.), *Minnesota symposium in child psychology (Vol. 16*, (pp. 41–81). Hillsdale, NJ: Erlbaum.

Stroufe, L. A. (1985). Longitudinal results in pre-school of infants classified in Ainsworth's "Strange Situation": Empathy, play, affect, and peer relations. Unpublished presentation to the Children's Service Clinical Conference on Attachment, Langley Porter Neuropsychiatric Institute, University of California, San Francisco.

Spitz, R. A. (1945). Hospitalism: An inquiry into the genesis of psychiatric conditions in early childhood. *The Psychoanalytic Study of the Child, 1*, 53–74.

Valliant, G. (1977). *Adaptation to life: How the best and the brightest came of age.* Boston: Little, Brown.

van der Kolk, B. A. (1989). The compulsion to repeat trauma: Reenactment, re-victimization, and masochism. *Psychiatric Clinics of North America*, *12*(2), 389–411.

van der Kolk, B. A., Perry, J. C., & Herman, J. L. (1991). Childhood origins of self-destructive behavior. *American Journal of Psychiatry*, *148*(12), 1665–1671.

Wachsman, L., Schuetz, S., & Chan L. S., (1989). What happens to babies exposed to phencyclidine (PCP) in utero? *American Journal of Drug and Alcohol Abuse*, *15*(1), 31–39.

Walker, E. S., Katon, W. J., Harrop-Griffiths, J., Holm, L., Russo, J., & Hickok, L. R. (1988). Relationship of chronic pelvic pain to psychiatric diagnosis and childhood sexual abuse. *American Journal of Psychiatry*, *145*, 75–80.

Weiss, R. S. (1991). The attachment bond in childhood and adulthood. In C. M. Parkes, J. Stevenson-Hinde, & P. Morris (Eds.), *Attachment across the life cycle* (pp. 93–114). London: Tavistock/Rutledge.

Wurtele, S. K., Kaplan, G. M., & Keairnes, M. (1990). Childhood sexual abuse among chronic pain patients. *Clinical Journal of Pain*, *6*, 110–113.

Chapter Seven

Psychosocial Vulnerability to Chronic Dysfunctional Pain: A Critical Review

Donald S. Ciccone and Veronica Lenzi

Fortunately, the vast majority of patients who sustain painful injuries recover spontaneously within a matter of weeks or months. For certain individuals, however, the onset of pain, whether of traumatic or insidious origin, marks the beginning of a slow but steady descent into permanent and total disability. We will refer to the constellation of symptoms associated with this decline in functioning as chronic dysfunctional pain (CDP). The presenting symptoms may include any or all of the following: avoidance of responsibility at work or at home; somatic preoccupation; over use of health care resources; inappropriate or exaggerated illness behavior; excessive inactivity; depression; and abuse of prescription medication. Efforts to provide a medical or purely organic explanation for CDP have met with repeated failure (Waddell, 1987). At the same time, there is mounting evidence that psychological or psychosocial variables are responsible for mediating many if not most of the symptoms associated with pain-related disabiliity (e.g., Cats-Baril & Frymoyer, 1991; Lancourt & Kettelhut, 1992).

If CDP is not the result of organic factors, then why do certain individuals become disabled following a painful injury while others who sustain comparable tissue damage either recover completely or continue to function despite the presence of pain? For those who accept the primacy of nonorganic factors in the etiology of CDP, this is a critical issue, and it is the one we attempt to address in this chapter.

Ideally, a psychological model of CDP should enable us to predict at the acute stage who will develop CDP and who will not. At a minimum, this model should identify salient risk factors or vulnerability markers. As noted previously, efforts to identify such factors have generally found nonorganic variables to have more predictive value than organic variables. Specifically, inappropriate illness behavior, premorbid stress, negative work appraisal, educational level, and perceived compensability have all demonstrated predictive utility in prospective studies using regression models to "predict" chronic disability (Cats-Baril & Frymoyer, 1991; Lancourt & Kettelhut, 1992). These same studies show that organic variables, such as restricted range of motion, neurological status, or imaging results, contribute little or no predictive information. There is empirical support, therefore, for the general assertion that nonorganic factors may effectively determine an indiviual's risk of chronicity following the onset of pain. Beyond stating that nonorganic factors are somehow involved in mediating treatment outcome, however, there is little else we can assert with confidence. At present, there is insufficient evidence to implicate a specific set of factors capable of identifying, at the acute stage, those individuals most likely to embark upon a chronic or protracted course.

Our goal in this chapter is to provide an overview of selected psychological or psychosocial variables that may be responsible for exacerbating the symptoms of acute injury. Rather than attempt a comprehensive review, we will focus instead on those few variables that have received empirical support and that lend themselves to theoretical interpretation. For example, the previously cited study by Lancourt and Kettelhut (1992) showed that patients with living arrangements lasting 7 years or longer tended to have a higher incidence of disability. While interesting, such findings are difficult if not impossible to interpret and we tend to overlook them in this review. Our discussion will also necessarily omit mention of potentially important factors about which relatively little is known. For example, Radanov, Dvorak, and Valach (1992) have documented the existence of subtle neuropsychological impairments assocated with hyperextension–hyperflexion (whiplash) injury. It may be that whiplash victims sustain undetected closed-head injuries that compromise their ability to regain premorbid function. At present, the incidence of brain injury among patients with chronic pain and its relationship, if any, to the symptoms of CDP is not known (Anderson, Kaplan, & Felsenthal, 1990). In a related vein, Flor, Schugens, and Birbaumer (1992) found that patients with chronic pain underestimated the extent to which their muscles were contracting relative to a group of healthy controls. Interestingly, impaired proprioception among the pain patients was not limited to the affected body part. The authors raised the possibility that failure to discriminate tension levels may lead to habitual overactivity and thus be a cause of chronic pain. Again, the relevance of this perceptual impairment, if indeed there is such an impairment, to the development of CDP has yet to be established by prospective research.

Within the constraints noted above, the following discussion will review the evidence that psychological or other nonorganic factors are implicated in causing or exacerbating disability following the onset of acute injury or illness. The pschological variables to be discussed fall into five broad categories: (1) premorbid psychiatric illness; (2) premorbid activity lvel; (3) cognitive dysfunction; (4) exposure to maladaptive (unhealthy) reward contingencies; and (5) premorbid trauma and/or prior illness.

Premorbid Psychiatric Illness

The relationship, if any, between premorbid psychiatric illness and chronic pain has yet to be established by well-controlled prospective research. There is, however, a retrospective study by Atkinson, Slater, Patterson, Grant, and Garfin (1991) that examines the prevalence of psychiatric illness among a sample of 100 male patients with chronic low back pain. Using a structured diagnostic interview, they compared the prevalence of psychiatric illness in the pain sample with an age-matched sample of healthy controls. In an effort to establish whether psychiatric illness preceded or followed the onset of pain, they used a matching procedure to "yoke" pain patients with controls of the same age. They then determined the frequency of psychiatric disorder among patients and age-matched controls up to the age at which the patient developed chronic pain. Based on such yoked comparisons, they found that alcohol-use disorders were more prevalent among pain patients than among controls before the age of pain onset. Specifically, 52.6% of pain patients who developed alcohol abuse or dependence did so before the onset of their pain. For pain-free patients, only 30.6% of those who developed an alcohol use disorder did so by the same age as did their yoked counterpart. Depressive and anxiety disorders were found to be more prevalent among pain patients than among controls, but when patients were matched using the yoking procedure to control for age of onset, only alcohol use disorders were found to reliably precede the development of chronic pain.

In one of the few prospective studies designed to identify psychological precursors of chronic pain, Dworkin, Hartstein, Rosner, Walther, Sweeney, and Brand (1992) found that heightened- state anxiety during the acute stage of herpes zoster (along with pain severity and disease conviction) predicted the likelihood of chronic pain. These investigators did not assess the prevalence of premorbid alcohol abuse in their patient sample, but one may speculate that patients with anxiety disorders are more likely to develop problems with alcohol use than those without anxiety. Taken together, therefore, the studies by Atkinson et al. and Dworkin et al. suggest a possible link between premorbid affect and risk of developing CDP. Obviously, such a conclusion is speculative in the absence of adequate prospective data. Although entitled a "prospective investigation," Dworkin et al. actually administered the anxiety questionnaire to patients after the onset of their acute pain. As a result, the data they obtained were not related to premorbid function, but rather reflected a post hoc response to the onset of herpes zoster.

Premorbid Activity Level

In an early uncontrolled study, Blumer and Heilbronn (1981) examined 234 patients who were seeking surgical treatment for intractable pain. They found that 41% of these patients had a history of frequent overtime hours and 63% said they were working before the age of 18. Based only on interview data and projective testing, they speculated that prior to the onset of pain, these patients had "performed in a slave-like manner, working and keeping active beyond average expectations at a pace they could not endure in order to be accepted and to atone" (p. 401). The possibility that excessive premorbid activity leads to chronic pain and disability was subsequently tested by Blumer and Heilbronn (1982) in a controlled retrospective study. They compared 129 patients with chronic pain (i.e., patients whose pain was found to have no "somatic basis") with 36 control patients who had been diagnosed as having rheumatoid arthritis. Both chronic pain patients and the controls rated their premorbid activity level as "more than average" (71% versus 72%, respectively). However, 35% of those in the chronic group claimed they had been working since childhood, whereas only 11% of those in the control group made this claim. Almost twice as many pain patients as controls indicated they had worked frequent overtime hours (50% versus 28%), and significantly fewer pain patients had taken vacations on a yearly basis (52% versus 78%).

In an effort to obtain a more reliable estimate of premorbid activity, VanHoudenhove, Stans, and Verstraeten (1987) used two different comparison groups to control for the possibility that memory for preinjury behavior is biased by a nonspecific "contrast" effect (i.e., patients who sustain a loss of function for any reason may recall their premorbid activity level as being higher than it actually was because of the contrast between their preinjury versus postinjury life-style). To evaluate this possibility, VanHoudenhove et al. administered a test of "action proneness" to: (1) 30 patients with chronic pain; (2) 30 patients with "organic" pathology (10 with paraplegia, 20 with MS); and (3) 30 patients who were hospitalized for psychiatric illness. A statistical comparison showed that patients with chronic pain reported significantly higher levels of premorbid activity than did either the "organic" or the psychiatric patients. If memory for premorbid behavior is influenced by a contrast effect, then organic patients should inflate their self report to the same extent as pain patients and we should not expect to see a difference (since loss of function was comparable for both groups). The fact that this did not occur makes it more difficult to attribute the reported hyperactivity of pain patients to biased recollection.

A recent study by Gamsa and Vikis-Freiberg (1991) provides additional evidence of premorbid hyperactivity among patients with chronic pain. Based on the earlier work of Blumer and Heilbronn (1981), they developed a questionnaire to assess so-called "pain prone" characteristics, including ergomania, or excessive work behavior. Specific items comprising the ergomania scale were: a history of early work onset, frequent overtime, and infrequent vacations. A comparison of 244 pain patients with 81 healthy controls revealed a significantly higher prevalence of ergomania among the patient population. The ergomania scale accounted for a significant amount of between-groups variance even after controlling for the effects of sex, occupational status, educational level, and other related variables.

Based on retrospective data, each of the foregoing studies has found evidence of premorbid hyperactivity among patients with CDP. A prospective study, however, reported by Murphy and Cornish (1984) seems to suggest quite a different pattern of premorbid behavior. These investigators administered a battery of psychological tests to a group of 48 male patients with "acute" low back pain and then monitored their progress for a period of 6 months to determine whether they recovered or became chronic. Among other findings, they reported that acute patients who became chronic had a lower premorbid activity level based on their responses to Scale 9 (Ma) on the Minnesota Miltiphasic Personality Inventory (MMPI). This scale is said to reflect a tendency toward overactivity or hypomania. Items on the scale appear to be somewhat heterogeneous but include the following: "It makes me impatient to have people ask my advice or otherwise interrupt me when I am working on something important"; "I have periods of such great restlessness that I cannot sit long in a chair." A discriminant function analysis revealed that patients who scored higher on Ma (i.e., had more hypomanic traits) were more likely to recover. While interesting, the results of the Murphy and Cornish study are difficult to interpret since it defined an acute patient as having "a presenting complaint of low back pain of less than 6 months duration." It is estimated that 40% to 50% of those seeking medical treatment for back pain show improvement within 1 week, and 90% are improved or recovered within 8 weeks (Steinberg, 1982). Those who continue to complain of pain after 3, 4, or 5 months may well be suspected of having a chronic problem. Murphy and Cornish do not specify how many of their "acute" patients actually had pain lasting longer than 3 months. If, as we suspect, many of the patients in their sample were actually chronic, then the entire logic of their design is invalidated and the results of the study are rendered meaningless. The likelihood that they failed to adequately sample from an acute-pain population is strengthened by the fact that 28 out of the 48 patients in their original sample were ultimately classified as chronic. The incidence of chronic back pain following an acute injury is widely estimated to be anywhere from 2% to 10% (Steinberg, 1982). The incidence in their sample was 28/48 or 58%. Although we may have good reason to question the data of Murphy and Cornish, this does not necessarily enhance our confidence in the retrospective data cited previously. It seems fair to state that the relationship, if any, between premorbid activity and chronic pain deserves further study and probably should be addressed in future prospective research.

Cognitive Dysfunction

According to social learning theory (Bandura, 1986), thinking or cognition lies at the root of all human endeavor. Accordingly, it has been suggested that cognitive events causally influence the development of many if not most of the symptoms associated with CDP (Ciccone & Grzesiak, 1984). It stands to reason that if cognitive theory is correct, then certain thought patterns or "cognitive errors" may increase the likelihood of becoming disabled following the onset of acute injury. Nevertheless, we are not aware of any prospective study that has examined the presence of irrational or distorted cognition in patients who subsequently became disabled by pain. We do know that patients with chronic pain tend to think irrationally about their symptoms and about life experiences in general (Lefebvre, 1981). However, the relationship, if any, betwen cognitive error and subsequent chronic pain is unclear. Obviously, irrational thought, in and of itself, in the absence of physical trauma or illness, does not increase one's risk of pain and disability. Individuals with chronic pain seem to perform about as well as individuals with no pain on a test of irrational thinking (see Table 1, Lefebvre, 1981).

In an effort to examine the relationship between cognitive distortion and disability, Smith, Follick, Ahern, and Adams (1986) administered the Sickness Impact Profile (SIP) and the Cognitive Error Questionnaire to a group of patients with chronic low-back pain. The former instrument is a self-report measure of physical impairment, while the latter is a test of irrational thinking developed by Lefebvre. Smith et al. (1986) found that severity of disability (on the SIP) was significantly correlated with "overgeneralized" thinking. The latter is a cognitive error involving the tendency to draw unwarranted inferences based on insufficient data. For example, if a patient has pain while performing a specific activity, he or she may erroneously conclude that all activities will similarly exacerbate pain. As a result of this thinking mistake, patients may come to avoid movement altogether and become excessively inactive. The fact that those patients who reported more disability were also those who tended to think in an overly generalized manner about pain suggests that cognitive errors of this kind may represent a potential vulnerability factor. Of course, the Smith et al. study was restricted to patients who already had chronic pain (the average duration of pain was over 4 years). A more convincing demonstration of vulnerability would require the administration of a cognitive error questionnaire at the acute stage of injury. Patients who scored high versus low on the overgeneralization measure could then be tracked over time to determine their respective rates of chronic disability.

A more recent study of cognitive dysfunction in patients with chronic pain has been reported by Riley, Ahern, and Follick (1988). These investigators developed a 15 item questionnaire designed to assess patient beliefs about the relationship between pain and functional impairment. Patients were asked to indicate their degree of agreement or disagreement with statements such as: "I can still be expected to fulfill my work and family responsibilities despite my pain." Riley et al. (1988) theorized that patients who attribute their physical impairment to pain may experience higher levels of disability than comparable patients who reject the idea that pain and disability are necessarily linked. In accordance with this expectation, they found that patients with higher scores on the Pain and Impairment Relationship Scale (PAIRS), who believed that pain was the cause of their physical impairment, were more likely to report higher levels of disability on the SIP. This correlation was statistically reliable even after partialing out that portion of the variance in SIP scores that could be accounted for by pain intensity ratings. Riley et al. (1988) point out that pain is not, in fact, a necessary cause of disability, since many pain patients increase their level of functional activity during treatment despite the presence of unrelenting pain. They further note that chronic pain, by definition, is intractable and that by linking functional impairment with pain relief, some patients may actually perpetuate disability as the result of a thinking error. By implication, this "error" may constitute a cognitive risk factor for disability. Although the relationship between PAIRS and subsequent disability has been replicated (Slater, Hall, Atkinson, and Garfin, 1991), prospective research has yet to establish the utility of any cognitive variable for identifying individuals at "risk" of disability.

In a related attempt to explain the cognitive causes of disability in a chronic pain population, Waddell, Newton, Henderson, Somerville, and Main (1993) developed a brief questionnaire (16 items) designed to assess patient beliefs about the impact of work and physical activity on their "medical" condition. The questionnaire is based on the notion that patients with chronic pain avoid work (and physical activity in general) because of their unfounded fear that activity causes increased pain and/or injury. Patients were asked to agree or disagree along a 7–point scale with statements such as: "I should not do my normal work with my present pain." Based on a sample of 142 patients, a hierarchical regression analysis was used to partition the variance associated with self-reported work loss in the preceding 12 months. Waddell et al. (1993) found that a subset of items reflecting "fear avoidance" beliefs explained 26% of the variance in the dependent measure. Only 5% of the variance could be accounted for by pain-severity ratings, and an additional 2% could be explained by the presence of depressive symptoms (as measured by the Zung Depression Inventory). While these results are interesting, it is entirely possible that so-called "fear avoidance" beliefs develop slowly over the course of chronic illness and play no role whatever in the etiology of CDP.

Beyond the obvious lack of prospective research, there may be a less obvious but equally difficult task confronting those who wish to identify cognitive risk factors. That task is deciding how to select and define the cognitive constructs they wish to study. The questionnaire developed by Riley et al. (1988), for example, is described as "tapping a singular construct." But even a cursory examination of the 15 items included in PAIRS reveals the presence of multiple thinking "errors," any one or all of which may elevate the patient's risk of disability. A number of items implicitly or explicitly endorse an external locus of control (Rotter, 1966). This is the belief that behavior is not governed by internal choices, but rather by external forces over which one has little or no control. The tendency to "externalize" in this manner is positively correlated with perceived pain (see Keefe & Williams, 1989) and may thus perpetuate inappropriate illness behavior in patients with CDP. Other items on the Pain and Impairment Relationship Scale suggest a tendency toward overgeneralizing (e.g., "I'll never be able to live as well as I did before pain"). By implication, many of the items reflect a tendency to misconstrue or misappraise the significance of pain, a tendency that may be linked to either somatizing or catastrophizing (Rosenteil & Keefe, 1983). None of these constructs are addressed in the Riley et al. study (1988), and thus their relevance or irrelevance to the construct under investigation is unclear. Before proposing that one or another cognitive variable may alter a patient's risk of disability, it seems essential to clearly define that variable by specifying how it relates or does not relate to other cognitive constructs. It may be useful to illustrate this point by using a concrete example. Dolce, Crocker, and Doleys (1986) have found that self-efficacy ratings correlate with likelihood of returning to work in a heterogeneous sample of chronic pain patients. But we already know (or at least suspect) that "overgeneralizing" leads to excessive inactivity and may perpetuate disability. Is it possible that perceived efficacy and overgeneralized thinking are related? This is indeed possible if patients jump to erroneous conclusions about efficacy based on incomplete or insufficient information. If so, which construct—efficacy or overgeneralizing—is more relevant to the assessment of risk status and how should we operationally define it?

A similar lack of clarity at the conceptual level makes it difficult to interpret the apparent relationship between "somatizing," on the one hand and increased risk of chronic disability, on the other. S. Dworkin, Wilson, & Massoth (see Chapter 2) report that patients who score high on the somatization scale of the SCL-90 tend to report higher levels of functional impairment than do patients who score low. But what exactly does it mean to say that a patient has a tendency to "somatize?" If somatizing is a risk factor, then how does it cause disability in an affected individual? The measure of somatizing used by S. Dworkin et al. (see Chapter 2) is limited to an assessment of affective distress. This is because they equate somatizing with "the tendency to report distress arising from perceived physical symptoms." This definition does not clarify the relationship between somatizing and other psychological variables that may be involved. For example, it has been suggested that certain individuals manifest physical rather than emotional symptoms in response to stressful life circumstances. For these individuals, the perception of threat might elicit pain or some other somatic response instead of the usual symptoms of depression and anxiety. Sifneos (1973) has suggested that the ability to label and/ or communicate affective experience may be restricted in patients with chronic pain or other psychosomatic illness. He uses the term "alexithymia" to describe this supposed disconnection between affect and self awareness. The inability to recognize or express negative emotion may thus manifest itself in a preference for somatic or physical symptoms. If it can be shown that emotional expression is indeed constrained in certain individuals by structural or linguistic factors, as the concept of alexithymia implies, then perhaps Dworkin's definition of somatization will need to be revised.

From a cognitive perspective, somatization may be defined by the specific beliefs or attitudes that cause the patient to focus on or misconstrue the meaning of physical sensation. Dworkin and Wilson (1992) acknowledge the role of cognitive factors in chronic pain, but they do not address the possibility that certain beliefs may predispose selected individuals to become "somatizers" or that somatizing itself may be defined as a set of specific beliefs about the meaning of pain. It may be useful, for example, to define somatizing as a tendency to misappraise or catastrophize negative sensation. Unwarranted inferences about the meaning of pain may be based on the (mistaken) assumption that all pain or discomfort is necessarily a threat to health or well being. These erroneous inferences could readily explain the presence of affective distress as measured by the SCL-90. In addition, muscle guarding, excessive inactivity, and unnecessary utilization of health-care services in somatizing patients could also be construed as consequences of this cognitive set. Of course, the use of concepts such as alexithymia or illogical thinking to "explain" somatization may or may not improve on the predictive utility of an SCL-90 test score. Nevertheless, an empirical correlation between psychological test scores and subsequent disability status does not in itself advance our understanding of vulnerability. It is our theoretical understanding of the "risk factor" in question that determines how we measure it and how it relates to other variables that may also predict risk status. A decision to measure somatization using an affective checklist (such as the SCL-90) means that we may overlook or fail to adequately investigate conceptually related variables (such as catastrophizing) that may also contribute to risk.

As noted previously, a prospective study of chronic herpes zoster pain by R. Dworkin et al. (1992) found that "disease conviction" as measured by the Illness Behavior Questionnaire (IBQ) was one of only three factors contributing unique variance to a discriminant function analysis. Patients who score high on the Disease Conviction scale of the IBQ are said to perceive any and all bodily sensations as symptomatic of serious illness. According to Pilowsky and Spence (1976), these patients cannot accept medical assurance that their symptoms are benign, and instead ardently amplify or otherwise distort the severity of their physical condition. Presumably, these are the same patients who Dworkin and Wilson (1992) (see Chapter 2) refer to as "somitizers." If so, then the prospective IBQ data reported by Dworkin et al. (1992) lend support to the suggestion by Dworkin and Wilson (based on retrospective SCL-90 data) that somatizing is indeed a possible risk factor for chronic pain. The fact that "fear avoidance" beliefs at least partially explain the extent of work loss in chronic back pain (Waddell et al., 1993) provides added support for the somatization hypothesis. Specifically, the Waddell finding means that "somatizing" or excessive apprehension about physical symptoms may result from a tendency to misconstrue or misappraise the significance of physical sensation. The resulting anxiety about pain or reinjury may perpetuate or even cause the prolonged disability associated with CDP. Of course, this hypothesis is purely speculative.

Exposure to Maladaptive Reward Contingencies

The operant model of chronic pain introduced by Fordyce, Fowler, Lehmann, and Delateur (1968) holds that maladaptive illness behavior is directly strengthened (i.e., its probability of occurrence is increased) by "unhealthy" reward contingencies in the environment. Thus the solicitous spouse who becomes more attentive following the onset of pain is described in operant terms as a reinforcing consequence of inappropriate pain behavior. In this way, environmental reward may influence the patient's risk of long-term disability. Alternatively, we may view illness behavior as the result of a conscious or unconscious choice on the part of the patient (Ciccone & Grzesiak, 1988). Such a cognitive interpretation is plausible in view of the fact that not all patients who are exposed to maladaptive reward contingencies actually develop inappropriate patterns of illness behavior. Regardless of the model we use to explain behavior, the mere availability of an environmental reward contingent on disability seems likely to increase the risk of CDP in selected individuals.

In particular, the opportunity to obtain financial reward may be, for some, a sufficient incentive to prolong or otherwise enhance the severity of an acute injury. Sander and Meyers (1984) reported that railroad workers who sustained painful back injuries lost, on average, 14.9 months from work when their injury was work-related versus 3.6 months when their injury was not work-related (i.e., when their injury was not compensable). Of course, injuries sustained on the job may or may not be comparable to those sustained off the job. In order to partially control for this possibility, Sander and Meyers created two matched groups of compensated versus noncompensated patients. The average age of the patients was similar and an effort was made to control for severity as well as type of injury. They found that patients who were compensated for time lost from work lost an average of 14.2 months, while those not compensated lost an average of 4.9. In addition, compensated patients who had spinal surgery lost an average of 9.3 months compared to only 4.4 for noncompensated patients who also had surgery. More recent studies by Greenough and Fraser (1989) and Jamison, Matt, and Parris (1988) have essentially replicated these findings. It appears that financial reward may either directly elicit disability behavior (according to operant theory) or, at the very least, enable such behavior by permitting injured workers to consciously or unconsciously avoid work.

An important methodological flaw in this research has been pointed out by Leavitt (1992). He argues that injured workers may be unable to resume premorbid job functions because of the physical demands associated with their job. He correctly points out that many patients who are disabled because of chronic back pain have a history of performing physically demanding work. Returning to work for these patients may entail an exacerbation of their symptoms or an increase in their risk of reinjury. Leavitt suggests that the probability of returning may thus depend more on the level of anticipated exertion and less on the availability of financial compensation. In order to test this theory, Leavitt compared patients injured on the job with patients injured off the job while controlling for "level of exertion" required at work. Contrary to his expectation, patients who were injured on the job were disabled for longer periods than patients injured off the job regardless of the physical exertion required by their premorbid occupation. For example, of the compensation patients who performed only sedentary work requiring no physical exertion, 27.8% remained disabled for more than a year. By contrast, of the noncompensation patients who performed sedentary work, only 10.2% were disabled for more than a year.

If compensation, in the absence of other mitigating factors, is an incentive for some patients to prolong disability, then we should expect a rapid resolution of symptoms once compensation is no longer available. In fact, even after their benefits are terminated, many patients continue to exhibit physical restrictions, and most do not return to their premorbid occupation or achieve their preinjury level of income (Linton, 1987; Mendelson, 1982). It may be that compensation for these patients is not a powerful disincentive at all; that is, most workers might not prolong disability simply for the sake of monetary gain. Instead, the effect of compensation may be to allow injured workers to avoid work that they perceive as unpleasant or that they find aversive in some way. Support for this possibility is provided in a study by Cats-Baril and Frymoyer (1991) that examines the utility of various organic and nonorganic factors in predicting disability following the onset of acute low-back pain. Using a prospective design, they administered a risk factor questionnaire to 250 study participants between the ages of 18–65 who reported a "new" episode of back pain. These individuals were then contacted 6 months later to determine their current disability or employment status (232 were reached for follow up). A discriminant-function analysis was used to identify a set of parsimonious predictors from the initial questionnaire. Those items achieving the highest levels of significance were reported to be "job characteristics—work status at the time the questionnaire was taken, work history, occupation, ratings on several aspects of job satisfaction, and satisfaction with retirement policies and benefits" (p. 606). Unfortunately, it is not possible to tell from Cats-Baril and Frymoyer's study precisely what dimensions of job satisfaction were actually assessed. Nevertheless, it appears that a negative perception of one's job may contribute to the risk of chronic disability following the onset of work-related injury.

This possibility is strengthened by the so-called Boeing study reported by Bigos et al. (1991). Over 3,000 workers who participated in the study were given a physical examination and asked to complete demographic, psychosocial, and workplace questionnaires. Each participant was followed for up to 4 years in an effort to identify risk factors associated with filing an acute back injury report at work. While the Boeing study is not directly relevant to our search for predictors of chronic disability, it is, nevertheless, one of the few long-term prospective studies involving the use of a work-satisfaction measure. The results showed that aside from a previous episode of back pain, the best predictors of acute back problems were "job enjoyment" and the ability to "communicate with peers." Considering these results and those of Cats-Baril and Frymoyer (1991) discussed previously, we now have tentative evidence that a negative perception of work not only increases the prospects of an acute work-related back injury, but also increases the probability that such an injury will become chronic.

Anyone who sustains a painful injury or develops chronic illness is likely to experience the socially rewarding consequences of illness behavior. These rewards are often provided by a well-meaning spouse, family member, friend, or health-care provider. A study by Flor, Kerns, and Turk (1987), for example, found that patients with a solicitous spouse were less active than comparable patients who were not socially "rewarded" by their spouse. There is also evidence that gender, marital status, and marital satisfaction may moderate the effects of social reward on patient behavior. Flor, Turk, and Rudy (1989) found that, in the case of male patients, a significant portion of the variance associated with pain intensity and pain interference ratings could be accounted for by solicitous spouse behavior. In the case of female patients, however, pain-impact scores could not be predicted by the presence of a solicitous spouse. When patients were categorized on the basis of marital satisfaction, pain-impact ratings could be predicted for all those who indicated an above average level of satisfaction (regardless of sex). Exposure to social reward following the onset of injury may, therefore, in the presence of certain moderating variables influence the likelihood of developing CDP.

Prexisting Illness or Trauma

The psychic effects of a painful injury or trauma may endure indefinitely and ultimately come to influence an individual's ability to cope with future adversity. Although this premise is widely accepted, there are, as yet, few studies documenting a relationship between preexisting trauma and impaired coping ability. For example, the possibility that preexisting trauma may adversely influence one's ability to cope with acute injury has not been shown. In addition, childhood experiences such as sexual, physical, or emotional abuse are routinely cited as risk factors for developing chronic pain as an adult but, in our opinion, with little empirical justification. In this section, we provide a highly selective review of the literature that purports to show a relationship between chronic pain and premorbid abuse or trauma.

The impetus for much of the research in this area is George Engel's (1959) classic article, " 'Psychogenic Pain' and the Pain-Prone Patient." This article makes a compelling case for the psychodynamic interpretation of chronic pain and continues to this day to stimulate research on the psychological origins of pain and disability. In a review written 25 years after the original paper, Roy (1985) summarizes Engel's position by stating that "a causal relationship is proposed between childhood abuse, introjection of pain, the association of pain with badness, and [the patient's] subsequent use of pain to expiate guilt" (p. 132). While this model of chronic pain is widely cited, it has yet to stimulate a precise or testable clinical hypothesis. In a relatively recent study, Adler, Zlot, Hurny, and Minder (1989) attempted to evaluate Engel's theory by determining the frequency of specific "developmental" factors among patients with so-called psychogenic versus organic pain. Specifically, they attempted to code interview data for the presence of childhood experiences such as: parents who were abusive toward one another; parents who were abusive toward the child; parents who were dominant or submissive; parents who were punitive or overcompensating; etc. Unfortunately, the authors failed to demonstrate that any of the above-mentioned experiences can be reliably coded from interview data or, for that matter, that any of these experiences can even be accurately recalled by the adult participants in their study. We do not believe the experimental comparisons between different groups of patients in the Adler et al. (1989) study warrant our discussion, since the assessment procedures used were so profoundly inadequate.

Even if we cannot readily establish the existence of specific parent–child interactions in the so-called pain-prone individual, we may be able to establish the presence or absence of other salient traumatic events. This is essentially the strategy adopted by Wurtele, Kaplan, and Keairnes (1990) in their study of childhood sexual abuse among chronic pain patients. They surveyed a group of 135 patients referred to a pain management program and found that 28% had been sexually abused by the age of 14. Unfortunately, in the absence of control group data it is impossible to evaluate the significance of this finding. For example, they cite a book by Russell (1986) that found that 32% of adult women in the general population have a history of sexual abuse. The fact that Wurtele et al. (1990) found a 39% incidence of sexual abuse among female chronic-pain patients may thus reflect the percentage of such abuse in the population at large.

A more convincing demonstration of the relationship between childhood sexual abuse and chronic pain is provided by Walker et al. (1988). These investigators used a structured interview to elicit sexual abuse histories from 25 women suffering from chronic pelvic pain (of 3 months duration or longer), and from a control group of 30 women undergoing gynecological examination either for infertility or possible tubal ligation. They found that 64% of women with chronic pelvic pain reported sexual abuse at or before the age of 14, while only 23% of women in the comparison group reported such abuse. The psychiatric interviewers were said to be unaware of the results of the patient's gynecological examination, but it is not clear whether they knew or did not know at the time of the interview whether the individual was a control or pain patient. Obviously, awareness of group membership, if indeed there was such awareness, might influence the manner in which data were collected. In any event, the rate of childhood sexual abuse among women with chronic pain in the Walker et al. (1988) study is double that reported by women in the population at large (Russell, 1986).

A second study by Walker, Katon, Neraas, Jemelka, and Massoth (1992) has replicated and extended the original findings. Again, they used a structured sexual assault interview with two groups of female patients. The first group was identical to the pelvic pain group in the earlier study, except that chronic pain was defined as lasting 6 months or longer (instead of 3 months). The second group of women were also treated at a university medical clinic but had no history of chronic pelvic pain. Again, patients with intractable pain were significantly more likely to report a history of childhood sexual abuse. Interestingly, 12 of 22 patients in the pain group experienced severe abuse, defined as "incest, rape, oral contact, or repeated fondling before age 14," compared to only 1 of 21 patients in the comparison group. The total number of patients included in the study was small, but the fact that an identical pattern of results was obtained across independent samples lends credibility to the notion that sexual assault in childhood may increase the risk of pelvic pain in adulthood for some women.

A recent study by Schofferman, Anderson, Hines, Smith, and White (1992) provides additional evidence that childhood experience and subsequent health status may be related. These investigators were interested in whether psychological trauma during childhood might influence the outcome of lumbar spine surgery in adulthood. Unfortunately, they elected to review patient charts retrospectively instead of obtaining evidence of abuse first hand through structured interviews or by some other means. The fact that those who coded the charts for childhood trauma were blind to spinal pathology and surgical outcome does not overcome the obvious limitatioins of a retrospective approach. In any event, Schofferman et al. (1992) coded 86 patient charts for the presence or absence of 5 different traumatic events (that had to occur before the patient was 22 years old). These events were: physical abuse—"intentional physical injury" by the child's primary caregiver; sexual abuse—exploitation or abuse of a child by an adult as a method of achieving sexual stimulation; substance abuse in a primary caregiver; abandonment–loss of a primary caregiver; and emotional neglect or abuse—primary caregiver is perceived as unavailable for emotional support or is excessively critical. It is apparent from these definitions that Schofferman et al. (1992) did not rely on precise criteria in their efforts to code the patient's childhood experience. Yet they state that each chart contained a "preoperative psychiatric assessment that addressed each risk factor" (p. 139). Given the vagueness of their definitions, it is difficult to imagine how the psychiatric record could be relied upon to systematically evaluate each of the childhood events under investigation. In addition, the authors do not provide a quantitative description of interrater reliability. They simply describe the reliability of their coding procedure as "excellent." As for outcome assessment, surgery was coded as a failure if the patient did not return to work within 12 months following a spinal fusion, or within 6 months following a discectomy.

The correlation reported by Schofferman et al. (1992) between the number of traumas sustained during childhood and the risk of surgical failure is essentially linear. For every additional childhood trauma reported there is a corresponding increase in the failure rate of surgery. Specifically, 95% of those patients who reported no childhood trauma had "successful" spinal surgery. This is compared with only 73% of those patients who reported one or two traumatic events. The rate of success falls to only 15% in the case of those who reported three or more traumatic experiences. These data raise the possibility that severe or multiple traumatic events during childhood might exert a cumulative (or additive) effect on the victim's health status as an adult. Of course, the limitations of the methodology used by Schofferman et al. (1992) render any such conclusion premature.

We should also emphasize that nominally identical traumatic events are not necessarily perceived as identical by trauma victims. For example, victims who appraise a "traumatic" event as catastrophic or who blame themselves for causing the event may experience different psychological sequelae than do victims who do not catastrophize or blame themselves. Thus despite being subjected to three or more childhood traumas, 15% of the patients interviewed by Schofferman et al. (1992) reported a successful surgical result. This suggests that future research may need to assess not only the occurrence of trauma but the victim's perception of it as well. We also know that the long-term effects of trauma are mediated to some extent by whether the victim is willing and/or able to discuss the event with another person. In a series of studies, Pennebaker et al. (Pennebaker, Barger, & Tiebout, 1989; Pennebaker & Susman, 1988) have shown that the incidence of stress-related illness among trauma victims is higher for those who keep the traumatic event secret. Similarly, Beutler, Engle, Oro-Beutler, Daldrup, and Meredith (1986) have argued that indivudals who are emotionally constricted or unable to express intense affect may deplete or otherwise suppress the body's production of endorphins (endogenous opioids) and thereby increase their vulnerability to chronic pain. While there is evidence that stress does indeed reduce the available supply of endorphins (Cohen, Pickar, & Dubois, 1983), there is no data linking the inhibition of affect following trauma to increased likelihood of CDP. Nevertheless, the possibility is raised that failure to disclose personal trauma or abuse may have long-term negative health consequences. Future efforts to identify psychological precursors of chronic pain may wish to explore this proposed link between trauma and emotional expression.

Aside from abuse inflicted by a cargiver or other adult, children may also be traumatized by serious illness or injury. The possibility that hospitalization during childhood might exert an adverse effect on one's health as an adult was investigated by Pilowsky, Bassett, Begg, and Thomas (1982). They interviewed 114 patients from a heterogeneous pain clinic population and requested information concerning childhood hospitalizations from birth to the age of 16. Two comparison groups were also included in the study, including 61 patients enrolled at a rheumatology clinic and 53 patients receiving psychiatric treatment for depression. They found that the frequency and duration of hospitalization for pain patients was significantly greater than that for rheumatology patients. It is interesting that there were no significant differences between pain patients and those receiving treatment for depression. Pilowsky, Bassett, Begg, and Thomas (1982) point out that exposure to an extended sick role is a learning experience that may sensitize children to the use of illness behavior as a coping mechanism. As adults they may be more apt than others (who have not been hospitalized) to use illness as a method of avoiding responsibility and/or exerting control over their environment.

Of course, the Pilowsky et al. (1982) data are equally consistent with a variety of other explanations, including the possibility that extended illness requiring hospitalization is especially likely to traumatize a child and thereby undermine his or her coping resources. Alternatively, children who are hospitalized may be prone to somatizing or hypochondriasis and simply continue in this vein when they become adults. It is even possible that children from dysfunctional families are more likely to be hospitalized than children from "normal" families (Apley &MacKeith, 1968). If this is true, then the underlying psychopathology of the family and the associated psychological abuse it inflicts on the child may readily account for the different rates of childhood hospitalization observed by Pilowsky et al. (1982). We should also note that none of the fore-going "explanations" is mutually exclusive and that a given indi-vidual may be influenced by one factor or by a combination of factors.

A Concluding Comment on the Psychosocial Origins of CDP

As yet, we have no reason to believe that psychological factors are routinely the cause of intractable pain in the absence of physical trauma or illness. There is, however, reason to believe that inappropriate illlness behavior following the onset of acute injury, the hall-mark of chronic pain, may be mediated by a variety of nonorganic factors. For example, we have seen that somatizing (Dworkin et al., chapter 2 in this volume; McCreary, Clark, Oakley, & Flack, 1992), overgeneralized thinking (Smith et al., 1986), fear avoidance be-liefs (Waddell et al., 1993), job disatisfaction (Cats-Baril & Fry-moyer, 1991), and a history of premorbid trauma (Schofferman et al., 1992) or premorbid illness (Pilowsky et al., 1982) may all be as-sociated with longer-lasting and more severe symptoms following the onset of an acute injury. Unfortunately, many of the studies we have just reviewed are based on retrospective (and possibly biased) self-report data and suffer from a variety of other metholological flaws (including the use of biased or unrepresentative samples, lack of appropriate controls, inadequate measurement procedures, an excessive number of predictor variables relative to sample size, etc.). As a result, there is no justification as yet for claiming that certain individuals develop chronic pain because of their premorbid experience or because of any other specific psychosocial event. Nev-ertheless, we have made the point elsewhere (Ciccone & Grzesiak, 1988) that many if not most of the symptoms of chronic pain are psychological in nature (e.g., excessive inactivity, avoidance behav-ior, depression, over utilization of health-care services, somatic anx-iety, muscle guarding, excessive or abnormal illness behavior, etc.). If we are correct in this assertion, then one should expect these psy-chological phenomena to be "caused" or influenced by psychologi-cal events and not by organic variables reflecting the presence or absence of objective tissue damage. In other words, psychological or psychosocial events should figure prominently in our search for the antecedents of chronic pain. It only makes sense to look for organic causes or antecedents if we believe the symptoms under investigation can be explained by the "medical model." As Waddell (1987) and others have argued, however, it is not plausible to attribute the symptoms of chronic pain to a purely physical lesion or to a biomedical disease process. Given the vast individual differences that often characterize how humans respond to similar injuries and the apparently psychological basis of much pain-related disability (Waddell, Bircher, Finlayson, & Main, 1984), we should expect nonorganic factors to be better predictors of disability than organic factors and, indeed, this seems to be the case (Lancourt & Kettelhut, 1992).

Although hardly definitive, the available research may serve to highlight promising leads or alert us to possible dead ends in our search for the psychological precursors of chronic pain. Before embarking on an expensive and time-consuming prospective study, preliminary findings derived from retrospective research may provide a rational basis for choosing predictor variables. It has been recognized for some time that prospective studies are the most elegant and probably the most appropriate way to identify potential "risk factors." The prospective approach entails an initial evaluation of the patient prior to symptom onset or, at a minimum, within days or weeks of onset, followed by prolonged observation and assessment for as long as necessary to isolate specific individual differences, psychological or otherwise, that discriminate those who regain function from those who do not. The extensive investment of both time and money required by prospective research may well explain the scarcity of these studies in the current pain literature (Sternbach & Timmermans, 1975).

The overall goal of prospective research should not be to simply predict the likelihood of chronic pain but rather to explain the psychological basis of nonorganic disability. Over the past few years, various demographic, anamnestic, and socioeconomic variables have been identified that seem to "predict" disability under certain circumatances (e.g., Burton & Tillotson, 1991; Volinn, Van Koevering, & Loeser, 1991) but, since they were not derived from a theoretical perspective, these variables often fail to explain the psychological phenomena underlying symptom formation. As a result, we believe the time has come to develop a heuristic model of chronicity that is not only consistent with current data (such as it is), but is firmly rooted in a more general theory of human behavior.

Such a model could serve as a basis for selecting predictor variables and provide a psychological context for interpreting the results of future prospective research.

References

Adler, R. H., Zlot, S., Hurny, C., & Minder, C. (1989). Engel's "Psychogenic pain and the pain-prone patient": A retrospective, controlled study. *Psychosomatic Medicine, 51*, 87–101.

Anderson, J. M., Kaplan, M. S., & Felsenthal, G. (1990). Brain injury obscured by chronic pain: A preliminary report. *Archives of Physical Medicine and Rehabilitation, 71*, 703–708.

Apley, J., & MacKeith, R. (1968). *The child and his symptoms, 2nd edition.* Oxford: Blackwell Scientific.

Atkinson, J. H., Slater, M. A., Patterson, T. L., Grant, I., & Garfin, S. R. (1991). Prevalence, onset, and risk of psychiatric disorders in men with chronic low back pain: A controlled study. *Pain, 45*, 111–121.

Bandura, A. (1986). *Social foundations of thought and action.* Englewood Cliffs, NJ: Prentice-Hall.

Beutler, L. E., Engle, D., Oro-Beutler, M. E., & Daldrup, R. and Meredith (1986). Inability to express intense affect: A common link between depression and pain? *Journal of Consulting and Clinical Psychology, 54*(6), 752–759.

Bigos, S. J., Battie, M. C., Spengler, D. M., Fisher, L. D., Fordyce, W. E., Hanson, T. H., Nachemson, A. L., & Wortley, M. D. (1991). A prospective study of work perceptions and psychosocial factors affecting the report of back injury. *Spine, 16*, 1–6.

Blumer, D., & Heilbronn, M. (1981). The pain-prone disorder: A clinical and psychological profile. *Psychosomatics, 22*(5), 395– 402.

Blumer, D., & Heilbronn, M. (1982). Chronic pain as a variant of depressive disease: The pain-prone disorder. *Journal of Nervous and Mental Disease, 170*(7), 381–406.

Burton, A. K., & Tillotson, K. M. Prediction of the clinical course of low-back trouble using multivariable models. (1991). *Spine, 16*(1), 7–14.

Cats-Baril, W. L., & Frymoyer, J. W. (1991). Identifying patients at risk of becoming disabled because of low-back pain. *Spine, 16*(6), 605–607.

Ciccone, D. S., & Grzesiak, R. C. (1984). Cognitive dimensions of chronic pain. *Social Science & Medicine, 19*, 1339–1345.

Ciccone, D. S., & Grzesiak, R. C. (1988). Cognitive therapy: An overview of theory and practice in chronic pain. In N.T. Lynch & S.V. Vasudevan (Eds.), *Persistent pain: Psychosocial assessment and intervention.* Boston: Kluwer Academic.

Cohen, M. R., Pickar, D., & Dubois, M. (1983). The role of the endogenous opioid system in the human stress response. *Psychiatric Clinics of North America, 6*, 457–471.

Dolce, J. J., Crocker, M. F., & Doleys, D. M. (1986). Prediction of outcome among chronic pain patients. *Behavioral Research and Therapy, 24*(3), 313–319.

Dworkin, R. H., Hartstein, G., Rosner, H. L., Walther, R. R., Sweeney, E. W., & Brand, L. (1992). A high-risk method for studying psychosocial antecedents of chronic pain: The prospective investigation of herpes zoster. *Journal of Abnormal Psychology,101*(1), 200–205.

Engel, G. L. (1959). "Psychogenic" pain and the pain-prone patient. *American Journal of Medicine, 26*, 899–918.

Flor, H., Kerns, R. D., & Turk, D. C. (1987). The Role of Spouse Reinforcement, Perceived Pain, and Activity Levels of Chronic Pain Patients. *Journal of Psychosomatic Research, 31*, 251–259.

Flor, H., Schugens, M. M., & Birbaumer, N. (1992). Discriminatiion of muscle tension in chronic pain patients and healthy controls. *Biofeedback and Self-Regulation, 17*(3), 165–177.

Flor, H., Turk, D. C., & Rudy, T. E. (1989). Relationship of pain impact and significant other reinforcement of pain behaviors: The mediating role of gender, marital status and marital satisfaction. *Pain, 38*, 45–50.

Fordyce, W. E., Fowler, R. S., Lehmann, J. F., & Delateur, B. J. (1968). Some implications of learning in problems of chronic pain. *Journal of Chronic Disease, 21*, 179–190.

Frymoyer, J. W., & Cats-Baril, W. (1987). Predictors of Low Back Pain Disability. *Clinical Orthopaedics and Related Research, 221*, 89–98.

Gamsa, A., & Vikis-Freiberg, V. (1991). Psychological events are both risk factors in, and consequences of, chronic pain. *Pain, 44*, 271–277.

Greenough, C. G., & Fraser, R. D. (1989). The effects of compensation on recovery from low back injury. *Spine, 14*, 947–955.

Jamison, R. N., Matt, D. A., & Parris, W. C. (1988). Treatment outcome in low back pain patients: Do compensation benefits make a difference? *Orthopedic Review, 17*, 1210–1215.

Keefe, F. J, & Williams, D. A. (1989). New directions in pain assessment and treatment. *Clinical Psychology Review, 9*, 549–568.

Lancourt, J., & Kettelhut, M. (1992). Predicting return to work for lower back pain patients receiving Worker's Compensation. *Spine, 17*(6), 629–640.

Leavitt, F. (1992). The physical exertion factor in compensable work injuries. *Spine, 17*(3), 307–310.

Lefebvre, M. F. (1981). Cognitive distortion and cognitive errors in depressed psychiatric and low back pain patients. *Journal of Consulting and Clinical Psychology, 49*(4), 517–525.

Linton, S. J. (1987). Chronic pain: The case for prevention. *Behavior Research & Therapy, 25*, 313–317.

McCreary, C. P., Clark, G. T., Oakley, M. E., & Flack, V. (1992). Predicting response to treatment for temporomandibular disorders. *Journal of Craniomandibular Disorders: Facial & Oral Pain, 6,* 161–170.

Mendelson, G. (1982). Not cured by a verdict-effect of legal settlement on compensation claimants. *Medical Journal of Australia, 2,* 132–134.

Murphy, K. A., & Cornish, R. D. (1984). Prediction of chronicity in acute low back pain. *Archives of Physical Medicine and Rehabilitation, 65,* 334–337.

Pennebaker, J. W., Barger, S. D., & Tiebout, J. (1989). Disclosure of traumas and health among holocaust survivors. *Psychosomatic Medicine, 51,* 577–589.

Pennebaker, J. W., & Susman, J. R. (1988). Disclosure of traumas and psychosomatic processes. *Med, 26*(3), 327–332.

Pilowsky, I., Bassett, D. L., Begg, M. W., & Thomas, P. G. (1982). Childhood hospitalization and chronic intractable pain in adults: A controlled retrospective study. *International Journal of Psychiatry in Medicine, 12*(1), 75–84.

Pilowsky, I., & Spence, N. D. (1976). Pain and illness behavior: A comparative study. *Journal of Psychosomatic Research, 20,* 131– 134.

Radanov, B. P., Dvorak, J., & Valach, L. (1992). Cognitive deficits in patients after soft tissue injury of the cervical spine. *Spine, 17*(2), 127–131.

Riley, J. F., Ahern, D. K., & Follick, M. J. (1988). Chronic pain and functional impairment: Assessing beliefs about their relationship. *Archives of Physical Medicine and Rehabilitation, 69,* 579–582.

Rosenteil, A. K., & Keefe, F. J. (1983). The use of coping strategies in chronic low back pain: Relationships to patient characteristics and current adjustment. *Pain, 17,* 33–44.

Rotter, J. B. (1966). Generalized expectancies for internal versus external control of reinforcement. *Psychological Monographs, 80* (Whole No. 609).

Roy, R. (1985). Engel's pain-prone disorder patient: 25 years after. *Psychotherapy and Psychosomatics, 43,* 126–135.

Russell, D. E. H. (1986). *The secret trauma: Incest in the lives of girls and women.* New York: Basic Books.

Sander, R. A., & Meyers, J. E. (1984). The relationship of disability to compensation status in railroad workers. *Spine, 11,* 141–143.

Schofferman, J., Anderson, D., Hines, R., Smith, G., & White, A. (1992). Childhood psychological trauma correlates with unsuccessful lumbar spine surgery. *Spine, 17*(6), 138–144.

Sifneos, P. E. (1973). The prevalence of "alexithymic" characteristics in psychosomatic patients. *Psychotherapy and Psychosomatics, 22,* 255–262.

Slater, M. A., Hall, H. F., Atkinson, J. H., & Garfin, S. R. (1991). Pain and impairment beliefs in chronic low back pain: Validation of the Pain and Impairment Relationship Scale (PAIRS). *Pain, 44,* 51–56.

Smith, T. W., Follick, M. J., Ahern, D. K., & Adams, A. (1986). Cognitive distortion and disability in chronic low back pain. *Cognitive Therapy and Research, 10*(2), 201–210.

Steinberg, G. G. (1982). Epidemiology of low back pain. In M. Stanton-Hicks & R. Boas (Eds.), *Chronic low back pain*. New York: Raven.

Sternbach, R. A., & Timmermans, G. (1975). Personality changes associated with reduction of pain. *Pain, 1*, 177–181.

VanHoudenhove, B., Stans, L., & Verstraeten, D. (1987). Is there a link between 'pain-proneness' and 'act-proneness'? *Pain, 29*, 113–117.

Volinn, E., Van Koevering, D., & Loeser, J. D. (1991). Back sprain in industry: The role of socioeconomic factors in chronicity. *Spine, 16*(5), 542–548.

Waddell, G. (1987). A new clinical model for the treatment of low back pain. *Spine, 12*, 632–644.

Waddell, G., Bircher, M., Finlayson, D., & Main, C. J. (1984). *British Medical Journal, 289*, 739–741.

Waddell, G., Newton, M., Henderson, I., Somerville, D., & Main, C. J. (1993). *Pain, 52*, 157–168.

Walker, E. A., Katon, W. J., Harrop-Griffiths, J., Holm, L., Russo, J., & Hickok, L. R. (1988). Relationship of chronic pelvic pain to psychiatric diagnoses and childhood sexual abuse. *American Journal of Psychiatry, 145*(1), 75–80.

Walker, E. A., Katon, W. J., Neraas, K., Jemelka, R. P., & Massoth, D. (1992). Dissociation in women with chronic pelvic pain. *American Journal of Psychiatry, 149*(4), 534–537.

Wurtele, S. K., Kaplan, G. M., & Keairnes, M. (1990). Childhood sexual abuse among chronic pain patients. *The Clinical Journal of Pain, 6*(2), 110–113.

Appendix

"Psychogenic" Pain and the Pain-Prone Patient

George L. Engel

In the past fifteen years, at two university medical centers, I have studied a large number of patients with pain. The great majority of these patients were seen in my role as a medical attending physician on the medical wards, teaching students and house officers, and as such included the usual variety of diagnosed and undiagnosed painful disorders ordinarily encountered on a medical service. A few patients were referred to me by colleagues who knew of my interest in pain. In addition, I have had random opportunities to observe the appearance and disappearance of pain during the course of psychoanalysis of patients with neuroses and psychosomatic disorders. The views about pain presented in this paper have evolved out of this clinical experience.

The Theoretical Problem

Pain is a cardinal manifestation of illness, and the relief of pain is probably the most common demand made by the patient upon the physician. In spite of the importance of pain, it is astonishing how little we understand pain, but how confident we are of our knowledge of pain. Perhaps familiarity breeds contempt. Every physician has his own personal experience with pain and it began long before he ever became a physician. This is in contrast to other complaints which we learn about only while studying medicine. The medical

student, when asked what pain is, feels at once that pain is something familiar, although he may have great difficulty defining it in
scientific terms. What he means is that he himself has experienced
pain and hence "knows" what pain is. When he is taught that
there are pain receptors, pain fibers, pain pathways, and a center
for pain perception, his concept of pain becomes scientific. To the
comfortable familiarity that comes from personal experience are
now added these simple "facts" and from this a relatively simple
concept of pain is constructed. Pain is the sensation which arises
when pain receptors are stimulated and it is transmitted via its
own fibers and pathways to the thalamus where it is perceived or
experienced. The more thoughtful student usually notes that whatever is transmitted from the periphery must also somehow or other
be perceived in consciousness, otherwise it is not pain. He may also
note that people seem to respond differently to whatever it is that
they perceive as pain. This insight then leads to the familiar formulation that pain has two components—the original sensation,
and the reaction to the sensation. There the matter usually rests.
When a patient complains of pain, it is taken for granted that pain
end organs somewhere in the body are being stimulated, presumably by a pathological process. That this often proves to be the case
provides repeated and comforting support to those who hold this
centripetal point of view. When no such explanation is found, it is
assumed that a pathological process is there nonetheless but simply has not yet been discovered. Rarely this to proves to be so. Or it
is postulated that something is affecting the nerves ("neuralgia"),
or the nerve pathways, or even the thalamus, producing so-called
"central" pain. If no other explanation is forthcoming, the patient
is told in one way or another that his pain is "imaginary," often
meaning that the physician does not believe it exists, in spite of the
most tangible evidence that the patient is suffering just as intensely as the person who has a visible and palpable painful lesion.
In more recent years the term "psychogenic" pain has come into
use and is generally applied by exclusion to those instances in
which no other cause of pain can be demonstrated. For many this is
a vague and mysterious concept since the commonly accepted concept of pain provides no room for such a notion. How can there be
pain if pain end organs are not being stimulated?

    I emphasize these points because unless you can relinquish the
notion that pain must originate in peripheral receptors and no-

where else, it is virtually impossible to understand what is referred to as "psychogenic" pain. Perhaps we need to ask first: What is pain? A definition of pain is elusive at best, if possible at all. As observers we cannot even recognize pain. Indeed, pain can only be experienced and for our information about pain we are totally dependent upon the report of the person experiencing it. As Szasz has pointed out, pain falls into the category of private data-experience which cannot be simultaneously shared and reported by anyone other than the person experiencing it (Szasz, 1957). It can only be reported. This is different from some varieties of experience, such as vision or hearing where what impinges on the sense organs can also be experienced by other observers and hence some consensus can be achieved as to what was seen or heard. Hence we have had no difficulty in discovering that occasionally persons may report seeing or hearing things in the absence of recognizable visual or auditory stimulation. One thinks at once of the hallucinations of psychotic people. However we should not overlook the fact that visual and auditory experiences in the absence of the corresponding peripheral stimulation are part of our daily life. Our dreams, for example, are predominantly and at times brilliantly visual in character-perhaps less often auditory. Some persons have a capacity for vivid visual and auditory imagery during the waking state. During complete sensory deprivation, including pitch darkness, there may be brilliant visual hallucinations (Solomon, Lieberman, Mendelson et al., 1957). A variety of chemicals, e.g., mescaline and lysergic acid, characteristically produce visual images (Osmond, 1957). Penfield has reported on the auditory experience in temporal lobe epilepsy and during direct brain stimulation (Penfield & Jasper, 1954). I make these points to emphasize that when it is possible to verify the presence or absence of a peripheral source of simulation in studying sensory experiences, we have no difficulty in identifying a host of examples in which no peripheral stimulation takes place and yet the person clearly experiences sensation. Arguing by analogy alone, I contend that the same must also hold true for pain.

What significance, then, are we to attach to the undoubted fact that there are pain pathways and that pain *can be* evoked by stimulation of parts of the body that are so innervated? Certainly it makes clear that in whatever manner we may conceptualize pain, one way in which it can be evoked is by appropriate stimulation of this peripheral sensory system. This does *not* justify the additional, usually inferred postulate that pain can *result only* from the stimulation of such pathways. But it does permit us to study and to identify characteristics of pain which are dependent on the neurophysiological characteristics of the peripheral system, an important consideration since this enables us to identify a pain process originating in muscle as compared to skin, for example. The peripheral distribution of pain-sensitive receptors has another importance in terms of how the individual's concept of pain develops. Pain belongs to the systems concerned with protecting the body from injury. We may assume that from birth on the individual builds up a library, so to speak, of pain experiences, originating from the variety of peripheral painful stimulations which he experiences during the course of his life. As we will show later, these are importantly concerned with the person's over-all development. Thus, from the developmental side we presume that the capacity to experience pain in the first place develops from numerous peripherally induced experiences but thereafter pain experience, like visual or auditory experience, may occur without the corresponding stimulation of the end organ.

There are still other reasons that compel us to question the purely centripetal concept of pain. We have already noted that only the sufferer knows whether or not he has pain and we may then ask: How does he know? Obviously *consciousness* and *attention* are necessary. Actually, the most successful technics for relieving pain, namely, general anesthesia and hypnosis, are not directed to pain *per se* but to consciousness and/or to attention. We know that the grievously wounded soldier in the heat of battle may experience no pain until the action is over.

Now, how do we know "pain" when it reaches our attention? We know it only by its quality and from this point on language fails us. It is completely impossible to describe pain accurately. We can describe it only in terms of experiences which evoke pain. Thus we may describe it as "sharp," thinking of a cut or a quick blow; or "dull," thinking of some slow pressure; as "burning," "tearing," or like a "pin-prick" or "toothache," and so forth. Obviously these are not descriptions of pain—these are descriptions of circumstances under which pain actually was experienced, or our imagination of how it would feel were something of this sort to be experienced. The man with a coronary occlusion may say it *feels like* his chest is being crushed, even though he may never have experienced actual compression of the chest and were he to experience it he would discover that it did not resemble his pain of coronary occlusion at all.

When we scrutinize more carefully the identifying quality of pain we note that it includes an affective tone. Pain is never neutral. It is usually unpleasant, but it may also be pleasant, if only in a relative sense. This effective quality brings pain into a very central position in terms of psychic development and function. Thus pain acquires special meanings for the individual as follows:

1. Pain warns of damage to or loss of parts of the body, and is part of the system for protection of the body from injury. It is, therefore, intimately concerned with learning about the environment and its dangers on the one hand, and about the body and its limitations on the other. We presume that what causes pain and the part that hurts are permanently registered in the central nervous system. We may, therefore, speak of "pain memories"* and of a "body pain image," the latter referring to parts of the body which have been sites of pain in the past.

2. In terms of development, pain is very much involved in human relationships (object relations). From infancy, pain leads to crying and to a response from the mother or some other close person. The association of pain → crying → comforting by a loved person → relief of pain, is an important determinant of tender love relations and helps to explain the "sweet pleasure" of pain. It is not the pain that is pleasurable, but the anticipation of reunion with a love object and the relief of the pain that are enjoyed. Certain individuals function as if the pain is worth the price.

3. Fairly early in childhood, pain and punishment become linked. Indeed, in many languages the two words spring from the same root. This establishes another kind of communication between the child and adults, namely, pain is inflicted when one is "bad." Pain thus not only may come to

*One is not able to re-experience a pain at will, but one may have memories about the pain. This is true of affects in general. Hence, the term "pain memories" refers to the ideational complexes, conscious and unconscious, associated with past pain experiences, stimulation of which may later give rise to pain. This pain is not the "old" pain anymore than the joy evoked by certain memories is the same joy that was felt on the occasion of the original joyous experience.

signal that one really is "bad," and thereby become a signal for guilt, but also pain may become an important medium for expiation of guilt. Some children as well as adults welcome pain if it means expiation and forgiveness and, hence, reunion with the loved one. If pain serves to relieve guilt, pleasure in a relative sense is again involved.

4. Pain also early becomes closely associated with aggression and power. The child quickly discovers the effects of inflicting pain on others and on himself. We will learn how by suffering pain one may control one's own aggression. The pleasure of the aggression is retained, but one's self is taken as the target.

5. Closely related to the preceding is the connection between pain and real, threatened, or fantasied loss of loved persons. Especially when there is also guilt for aggressive feelings toward such persons, pain may provide a psychic means of expiation. Further, as Szasz points out, the patient succeeds in reducing the feeling of loss by experiencing a pain in his own body which he then substitutes for the lost person (1956). He suffers more from the pain than the loss, so to speak. Later, we will see how the patient's ideas of pain actually or presumably experienced by the lost person will determine the location of the patient's pain. The psychic logic of this is revealed in our language when we speak of a "painful loss."

6. Pain may also be associated with sexual feelings. We know that at the height of sexual excitement pain may not only be mutually inflicted but actually enjoyed. When this becomes the dominant feature of the sexual activity, we recognize it as a perversion, sado-masochism. We will also discover some persons who prefer to experience pain rather than have sexual experience, the latter existing only at the level of unconsciousness fantasy.

When we examine the full gamut of circumstances, from the simple peripheral stimulus to the complex psychological components, we must acknowledge that pain in final analysis is a psychic phenomenon. The two-component concept of pain, which speaks of the pain sensation and the reaction to pain, is misleading because it implies that pain can originate only from a "pain" receptor.

Gooddy goes so far as to say: "There can be no pathways nor nerve endings for *pain*. The notion of pathways for pain is but a figment of the observer's mind" (1957). Instead he suggests that disordered patterns (rate, amplitude, time, and space) in nerves or neural centers provide the neurophysiological conditions which may be experienced as pain, but they do not by themselves account for pain. Certain characteristics of the impulse patterns may influence the quality of pain, but they will not in themselves determine that it be pain. This certainly is consistent with the clinical observation that one can identify qualities associated with colic, for example, as differentiated from a toothache, qualities which arise from the properties of the particular anatomical system giving rise to the disordered impulse patterns. Thus such patterns originating in the periphery contribute certain qualities to the pain and determine where the patient locates the pain, but the total pain experienced is always a psychic phenomenon.

This brings us then to "psychogenic" pain. While the pain experience is only and always a psychic phenomenon, it is nonetheless of both practical and theoretical importance to know whether or not what is being experienced as pain includes disordered patterns originating in nerve endings, just as we need to know whether or not a visual experience originated from light waves striking the retina. But the fact of a peripheral process does not necessarily mean pain, for we know that pathological changes may be associated with the most excruciating pain in one person and with little or no pain in another. By hypnosis, or with placebos, we may eliminate or induce pain without modifying to the slightest the nature of the pathological lesion (Rosen, 1951; Beecher, 1956). The practical clinical problem really has to do with how the individual experiences pain. Clinical observation reveals that there are people who seem to experience pain with unusual intensity and frequency. With peripheral lesions they seem to suffer more pain than most people do, but often they suffer pain without any peripheral process. Among such patients the presence or absence of a peripheral disorder is not well correlated with the presence or absence of pain. Indeed we often find that the discovery of the lesion and its removal or cure does not alleviate the pain, which may persist or even recur at a later date. In other words, there are certain individuals, whom we shall call "pain-prone," among whom psychic factors play the primary role in the genesis of pain, in the absence as well as in the presence of peripheral lesions.

Clinical psychologic studies of many pain-prone persons have by now provided us with a fairly good understanding of the determinants of this susceptibility to suffer pain (Szasz, 1956; Breuer & Freud, 1895/1955; Schilder, 1935; Engel 1951; Rangell, 1953; Kolb, 1954; Hart, 1957). The key comes through understanding how pain may yield pleasure. It is pleasure in a relative sense, that is, in place of something even more distressing. Beginning from a primitive protective system, pain evolves into a complex psychic mechanism, part of the system whereby man maintains himself in his environment. Both as a warning system and as a mechanism of defense, pain helps to avoid or ward off even more unpleasant feeling states or experiences and may even offer the means whereby certain gratifications can be achieved, albeit at a price. If we can understand this adaptive role of pain in the psychic economy, we can begin to comprehend how it is that certain persons actually seek pain, even to the extent of creating it as a purely psychic experience if no peripheral stimulus is available to evoke it.

The Clinical Problem

Let us now examine pain in terms of the problem as it is actually encountered by the physician, namely, a patient seeks medical aid because he is suffering from pain. I propose that we approach each patient with the following questions in mind:

1. Are there pathological processes affecting nerve endings and leading to disordered patterns in nerve pathways which are being experienced as pain?
2. If such processes are present, can the character of the pain experience reported by the patient be fully, partially, or not at all accounted for by the distinctive characteristics of the peripheral pathological process?
3. How are psychological processes operating to determine the ultimate character of the pain experience for the patient and the manner of its communication to the physician?

All three questions are pertinent with every patient, although circumstances as well as patients differ in respect to how much attention each question requires before our problem is solved. They acknowledge the principle that a peripheral factor may or may not be operating and that when it is operating it may not fully account for the pain experience. Further, they permit us to explore in more practical clinical terms the precise criteria which should enable us to make accurate interpretations. For example, if a man complains of epigastric pain, not a normal gastrointestinal x-ray series nor one showing some irritability of the duodenal cap will, by itself, provide the explanation for the pain. The patient may or may not have a duodenal ulcer, and if he has a duodenal ulcer this may or may not account for the pain which he experiences. When we examine what is called the typical "ulcer pain" we realize that there are distinctive characteristics of the pain associated with duodenal ulcer which we can recognize as the qualities conferred upon the total pain experience by the type of the disordered impulses arising in the nerve endings in the region of the ulcer. It is these qualities which permit us to identify duodenal ulcer as compared to biliary colic. Our first concern, then, must be with how the patient describes his pain.

The Description of the Pain

The Peripheral Signature

The relatively good concordance among individuals as to the kinds of pain associated with particular pathological processes gives us our first clue as to what differentiates the peripheral contribution to pain experience from the rest of the pain experience. Gooddy spoke of "disordered patterns," referring to rate, amplitude, time, and space, and we immediately recognize that what enables us to identify a particular pain experience as being associated with myocardial ischemia, or renal colic, or a perirectal abscess, or a bone metastasis, concerns how the specific anatomic and physiologic characteristics of the diseased part gives rise to these disordered "patterns" (1957). Wolff's meticulous study and demonstration of the varieties of pain evoked by stimulation of various parts of the head provides an excellent demonstration of the consistency of the signature conferred on the pain experience by anatomical and physiological factors (1948). With a stone in the ureter, we can predict with a high degree of confidence where the patient will locate the pain and we will recognize in the colicky character of the pain the rhythmic contractions of the ureter in its attempt to pass the stone. Further, once we understand the anatomy and physiology of the structure involved we can also predict that certain movements, postures and behaviors of the patient are chosen because they are associated with pain amelioration, while others are avoided because they are associated with the intensification of the pain.* While this is common knowledge, I stress it because the precise elucidation of such correlations between anatomical and physiological characteristics on the one hand, and pain experience on the other hand, provides the most certain evidence that processes originating in the periphery are initiating a particular pain experience. Conversely, deviation from these understandable anatomical and physiological principles should immediately caution the physician that peripheral disordered patterns play no role or their influence is being obscured by other factors. The patient, for example, with acute myocardial infarction who continues to experience the same pain unremittingly for a week arouses our suspicion. Does this indicate a further extension of the infarct? This is an unlikely possibility and would have to be established by means other than the pain itself. Could it be that pain that originated in relationship to the myocardial infarct now has established an existence independent of the changes taking place in the myocardium? Finally, could it be that the pain never was related to the myocardial infarct, but rather to something else which again may or may not be affecting nerve endings? The incongruity between the pain characteristics as described by the patient and the known pathophysiological and pathoanatomical processes is in itself sufficient grounds to question the accuracy of the interpretation which explains all on the presence of the allegedly demonstrated peripheral disorder. Here I would warn especially against the commonplace practice of describing such situations simply in terms of the pain being "atypical."

The Individual Psychic Signature

As we listen to the patient's account of his pain, we first attempt to detect and identify pain qualities associated with stimuli arising from the periphery, as just described. All the other features of the pain description are understandable in terms of what we might call the individual's "psychic signature," as contrasted to the "periph-

*In the two person field we may also note that certain movements, postures and behaviors are utilized by the patient with pain because of their value in communicating to others the need for help.

eral signature." What are some of the varieties of pain description that are not understandable in terms of a peripheral process, even when the latter is present? I have already mentioned discrepancies in respect to what would be predicted from anatomy and physiology. We need to pay attention to pain location in terms of the patient's concept of his body image as contrasted to pain location determined by the distribution of nerves. For example, the patient who locates his pain in the region of the left nipple or the apex beat may at some point indicate concern about heart disease. The doctor should consider the possibility that some idea about heart disease accounts for the location of the pain, although not for the pain itself, rather than the pain giving rise to the idea of the heart disease. Actually, patients with heart pain often prefer to explain the pain on the basis of something non cardiac, such as indigestion.

Patient's private concepts of how their bodies function may influence their description of pain. For example, the person who entertains an autointoxication theory may get pain relief from cathartics or colonic irrigations, such relief not indicating in any way colonic disease. The intensity of pain reported by patients is a highly individual matter. Clinical experience is a useful guide but, in general, gross deviations in direction inform us more of the psychic state of the individual than of the existence or nature of a peripheral lesion. Libman's test for pain sensitivity by styloid pressure is a useful way of evaluating quickly how a patient deals with a painful peripheral stimulation (Libman, 1934).

In general, the more complex the ideation and the imagery involved in the pain description, the more complex are the psychic processes involved in the final pain experience. In part this is a matter of reality testing. When the pain experience is initiated from the periphery and this is the primary factor responsible for its presence, and when the function of the pain is to signal to the patient damage or injury to a part of his body and nothing else, the pain description is likely to be economical and relatively uncomplicated. Terms such as "sharp," "dull," "aching," "throbbing," and the like are relatively easily applied and the relationship to physiological processes relatively easily identified by the patient. On the other hand, vague descriptions as well as more elaborate imagery are reflections of the degree to which the pain is entering in psychic function in a more complicated fashion, now serving purposes far beyond the simple nociceptive function. While the patient almost always initially presents his complaint as a pain, an ache, a headache, a backache or some such symptom, request for elaboration will sometimes, but not necessarily, bring out a vague description, as "a sensation," "an unpleasant feeling," "I just can't describe it"; or descriptions such as "being jabbed with an icepick," "burning like red-hot coal," "bruised and torn," "like my face is being eaten up," "electric shocks burning me," and "just too horrible to describe." Or "headache" may become "a sort of pressure as if the top of my head would come off." A backache may become "a pulling or drawing as if the cords of my back were being pulled at." Sensations described as boring, gnawing, biting, penetrating, crawling, twisting, and tearing are particularly meaningful. Now these varieties of description are extremely valuable in identifying the presence or absence of a peripheral process. In general, however, while we can be fairly confident of a peripheral lesion when the description is not only crisp and economical but also concordant with anatomical and physiological processes, we cannot conclude that the patient who gives us the more complex, the vague, or the vivid type of description does not have a peripheral lesion. Such descriptions reflect the characteristics of the individual, and if he is suffering from a peripheral lesion, the disordered patterns arising from it are subjected to the most complex psychic distortion and elaboration so that at times the peripheral qualities may be totally obscured.

This now brings us to explore *who* are the patients disposed to use pain in this fashion and under what circumstances do they do so. For convenience, we shall refer to them as the "pain-prone patients."

The Pain-Prone Patients

For the most part these patients repeatedly or chronically suffer from one or another painful disability, sometimes with and sometimes without any recognizable peripheral change. There are also patients who may have only a single or occasional episode of pain, among whom essentially the same psychic mechanisms are operative. Such patients by no means constitute a homogeneous group and yet they have many features in common. By recognizing and understanding the clinical expressions of the psychodynamic processes underlying this type of psychic function of pain, the physician will be able to recognize the patient who uses pain in this fashion and hence more correctly interpret each pain experience for which he is consulted.

The Choice of Pain as Symptom: Pain as punishment

I mention this component first because clinical observation leads me to conclude that guilt, conscious or unconscious, is an invariable factor in the choice of pain as the symptom, as compared to other types of body sensations. Clinically, we should expect to find a long-term background of guilt and/or an immediate guilt-provoking situation precipitating pain. The clinical characteristics of the chronically guilt-ridden person are not difficult to recognize, if one appreciates the role of penitence, atonement, self-denial, and self-depreciation as means of self-inflicted punishment to ease the feeling of guilt. The patient who uses pain as a means of self-punishment and atonement almost always manifests other psychological and behavioral devices that serve the same purpose, and their recognition will alert the physician to the likelihood that this patient is indeed using pain in this fashion.

Some of these individuals are chronically depressive, pessimistic, and gloomy people whose guilty, self-depreciating attitudes are readily apparent from the moment they walk into your office. They seem to have had no joy or enthusiasm for life and, indeed, some seem to have suffered the most extraordinary number and variety of defeats, humiliations, and unpleasant experiences. You may first be inclined to pass this off as a consequence of the pain they are suffering or as just a matter of bad luck. But it quickly becomes apparent that many of these difficult situations have been solicited by the patient or simply not avoided. They drift into situations or submit to relationships in which they are hurt, beaten, defeated, humiliated and, to our astonishment, seem not to learn from experience; for no sooner out of one bad spot they are in another in spite of the most obvious danger signals. At the same time they conspicuously fail to exploit situations that should lead to successes and, indeed, when success is thrust upon them they do badly. This provides the clearest proof that these characteristics are not the result of the pain, for we note often that it is just when life is treating them worst, when circumstances are the hardest that their physical health is likely to be at its best and they are free of pain. Paradoxically, when things improve, when success is imminent, then a painful symptom may develop. Unconsciously they do not believe that they deserve success or happiness and feel that they must pay a price for it. A common kind of statement is, "When I was having such a hard time, I felt good; but now, just when I should be able finally to enjoy myself, this terrible pain has to come." Even though they complain of the pain, for them the pain is almost a comfort or an old friend. It is an adjustment, a way of adaptation acquired through psychic experience. We are often struck by the disparity between the intensity of the pain and suffering they describe and their general appearance of well-being. Some patients may describe a terrible pain with so little evidence of current suffering that you may be surprised to discover that they are speaking of a present pain. This stoical behavior may express the need to see oneself and be seen as a martyr who tolerates suffering. Other patients display intense suffering, behavior which also has psychic determinants, including a need to appear as the suffering person, to be pitied or to be succored. Some patients seem to experience a secret joy in their pain while others appear literally to be persecuted by it. Many of these patients are unusually tolerant of pain inflicted upon them by nature or by the physician in the course of examination and treatment. In their histories we discover an extraordinary number of injuries and operations and more than the usual number of painful illnesses and pains, the latter usually described in medical jargon as "pleurisy," "kidney attacks," "sinus," "lumbago," "appendicitis," and the like. Careful history will usually render doubtful that such terms actually correspond with the diagnosis in more than a few instances. We soon realize that what many of the patients solicit from us is the infliction of further pain, usually in the form of surgery or painful diagnostic or therapeutic measures. Treatment that is not painful or a hardship may be rejected. Physicians may be surprised at how well these patients tolerate painful procedures. Indeed, the patient who is very fearful of such painful procedures is not likely to be found among this group at all.

The following cases are illustrative:

A 61-year-old man had suffered intense pain intermittently for 25 years in the region of the right ear. This pain had lasted for several days at a time and was described as "raw and burning." The patient's mother had died when he was 7½ years old. His father and stepmother had treated him harshly, and "boxing the ears" was a frequent punishment from both, a procedure to which he had submitted passively, although his younger brother had not. Characteristic of this man was that he had allowed himself to be struck by his father until his 21st birthday, feeling that he had no right to protest until he was legally an adult. However, he did not leave home until he was 26 years old and up to that time had contributed the major share of his earnings to his father. Face pain began about this time.

Although of superior intelligence, he had done heavy manual labor for many years. Later he had gone into business with a partner. The business was a success, but his partner had soon cheated him of all the profits and he had ended up losing everything. Like other events in his life, he had accepted this without a struggle.

Six years before examination, he had suffered a myocardial infarction and since then had experienced severe angina pectoris decubitus. The face pain became less severe from that time on.

A 53-year-old unmarried school teacher had had severe dysmenorrhea and headaches since the age of 18. At various times in her life she had had severe pains in her head, cheeks, teeth, abdomen, back, legs, and hips. The low back pain had been described as "like a raging toothache-sometimes like something is moving or crawling down my legs." She described a fantastic career of suffering, of which the following sequence is typical:

She had worked hard for almost 30 years, depriving herself of all comforts in order to build herself a house in which to retire. In the meantime she lived with an old woman who suffered from senile dementia and who made excessive demands. Finally the long-awaited day arrived and she moved into her new home. She soon began to feel guilty enjoying this all by herself, so she advertised for a roomer. She took in a young couple with two small children who soon spread out to occupy the whole house, the patient retiring to a single bedroom. When the new tenants complained that she interfered with their privacy, she had obligingly moved out, sold them the furniture at a loss, rented them the house for a ridiculously small sum and had returned to live with the senile lady.

With many of these patients we will be struck by the dramatic fashion in which they describe both the hardships of their lives and the extent of their suffering from pain, illness, and the slings and arrows of misfortune. Indeed, this very dramatic quality and the relish with which they recount the story, often an almost unbelievable one, should immediately alert the physician that this is a person for whom pain and suffering are unconscious sources of gratification.

A 44-year-old woman had a host of painful symptoms beginning in adolescence. At various times they included "appendicitis," "arthritis," "pleurisy," "kidney colic," "heart" pain, face pain, back pain, headaches, and pains in the extremities. She had had 14 major and minor operations and at least 5 painful injuries. Everything in her life was described in dramatic terms. The patient's relation to her mother had been a very ambivalent one, while towards her father she had felt most affectionate as a child. She had especially enjoyed resting her face on his shoulder. She recalled an occasion when she was 12 years old when her mother had had severe pain in the face due to a tooth infection. Although she was extremely frightened of the dark, she ran a considerable distance at night to get a doctor.

Early in childhood she felt her mother favored her four siblings. She deliberately provoked her mother by misbehaving and when her father came home from work she expected to be punished and indeed often was. This was actually a pleasurable experience because, after the spanking, her father would hold her on his lap and fondle her. She had many fears in childhood and would find these an excuse to jump into her father's bed for comfort. When she first began to menstruate she thought she was bleeding to death. When she was 22 years old she married a boy she hardly knew and her life with him was a nightmare. They lived with his mother who treated her as a servant. He drank, beat her, and openly brought prostitutes to the house and required his wife to wait on them. Occasionally she would leave her husband for a few months at a time but she always returned. At these times she lived with her well-to-do physician brother and his wife where she functioned essentially as a servant. When her father and later her mother became ill, she undertook the complete responsibility of their care.

Her father died in her arms when she was 30. Following his death the mother became depressed, and this depression lasted several years. The patient undertook her care and never left her alone. The first and only time the patient went out, her mother took the opportunity to commit suicide by throwing herself in front of a train. The body was badly mutilated and no one was permitted to see it. The patient repeatedly attempted to reassure herself that her mother's face had escaped mutilation. After her mother's death she finally brought herself to divorce her husband. At the age of 40 she married a 60-year-old man. Commenting on this marriage, the patient stated that she would be content to settle for 10 years of happiness. She called her husband "Daddy." No sooner had she entered what she called the first happy period in her life, when she quarreled with her sister-in-law and physician brother. Then the face pain developed which already had robbed her of the first 4 of her hoped-for 10 years of happiness.

The Development and Backgrounds of the Pain-Vulnerable Patients

For practical clinical purposes it is usually not necessary to elucidate all the factors predisposing to these developments. Suffice it to say that we often find that aggression, suffering and pain played an important role in early family relationship. These may include:

1. Parents, one or both of whom were physically or verbally abusive to each other and/or to the child.
2. One brutal parent and one submissive parent, the former sometimes an alcoholic father.
3. A parent who punished frequently but then suffered remorse and overcompensated with a rare display of affection, so that the child became accustomed to the sequence: pain and suffering gain love.
4. A parent who was cold and distant but who responded more when the child was ill or suffering pain, even to the point that the child invited injury to elicit a response from the parent.
5. The child who had a parent or other close figure who suf-

fered illness or pain for which he came to feel in some way responsible and guilty, most commonly because of aggressive impulses, acts, or fantasies.

6. The child who was aggressive or hurting until some event suddenly forced an abandonment of such behavior, usually with much guilt.

7. The child who deflected the aggression of a parent away from the other parent or a sibling onto himself, usually an early manifestation of guilt.

Some of these backgrounds are illustrated in the following excerpts of the histories of pain-prone patients. It is consistent with their psychological characteristics that these patients readily provide the physician with such information if only he indicates his interest to hear it. This eagerness to tell of such distressing life experiences is in itself of diagnostic value, and it is not of crucial importance whether such descriptions are factual or fanciful. In event, the fact and manner of telling betrays the wish of the patient to present himself as long-suffering and abused.

A 32-year-old married woman had cruel, impulsive parents. The father was a chronic alcoholic and the mother unpredictable and sadistic. She had vivid memories of being hit hard across the face and back by both parents. Mother would slap her face suddenly and without warning as insurance against future misdeeds. When the patient was 7, all of mother's teeth were extracted; the patient remembers the severe face pain suffered by the mother.

A 34-year-old married woman witnessed the death, by accidental burning, of her 2-year-old sister when she was 5. This little girl's clothes caught fire from a wood stove and her face was badly burned. Later, the parents separated and she was placed with an older couple. The foster mother frequently beat her about the face and head and pulled her hair. The patient said, "I often think of her when I have my pains."

A 27-year-old married mother had pain in the head, face, and eyes. As a child she frequently witnessed her brutal, alcoholic father slap her mother across the face. Her sister, 7 years younger, was born blind in one eye. The patient blamed the father for this and also accused him of preventing the girl from receiving proper medical attention. She herself undertook to obtain this care for her sister at the expense of great personal hardship.

A 41-year-old unmarried woman, a school teacher, had severe sharp pain involving the entire left half of the face and head. Since childhood she had always maintained the strictest control over the expression of any aggression. As a child, however, she had had a reputation of being a little "spitfire." This period came to a close when, in a fit of anger, she threw a pair of scissors which stuck in the left cheek of her little cousin. The mother warned her that retaliation in kind would befall little girls who throw things and put people's eyes out. From that time on she never actively expressed aggression externally.

Alternating with the face pain had been back pain. When she was 16 her father was killed in a mine accident. That day he had awakened with a backache and although his wife urged him to stay home and rest, he went to work and as a consequence was killed.

Under What Circumstances Does the Pain Occur?

Many of these people have had repeated episodes of pain, so that this question has two aspects: When did the patient first have pain, and when did each episode occur? Quite a number have their first significant painful syndromes in adolescence. This is especially so among women patients whose story may begin with painful menarche, dysmenorrhea, or headaches, especially premenstrual. A very important clinical finding is the history of "appendicitis" and appendectomy. These episodes do not fit the usual clinical picture of acute appendicitis, but usually involve chronic or intermittent abdominal pain of quite varied nature and severity, sometimes associated with a variety of other symptoms. Such attacks usually begin in the age range 14 to 18 years, eventually leading to appendectomy. When surgical records are available we find the appendix reported as "normal" or "chronic appendicitis." Curiously, this pain usually disappears after surgery, although it may soon be replaced by other pains often related by the patient and some physicians to the scar or to adhesions. This "appendix" syndrome is much more common among girls than boys and its presence in the past history provides a valuable clue for the interpretation of later pains (Eisele, Slee, & Hoffman, 1956).

The onset of pain syndromes in adolescence also reflects the important psychological changes occurring in this period of life, and especially the sexual conflicts that may be involved in the genesis of pain. Both guilt about sexual impulses and an unconscious sadomasochistic concept of sex are important. Pain may occur in lieu of or may prevent sexual activity, and hence under circumstances in which sexual impulses might be aroused, in fact or in fantasy. Frigidity, dyspareunia, and varieties of impotence are common accompaniments. Or the patient may enjoy some sexual pleasure if he is hurt (masochism). Along these same lines we may discover painful, mutilating, and destructive concepts of pregnancy and labor, among men as well as among women.

We may now consider some of the circumstances under which individual episodes of pain may occur, remembering that this may also include pain precipitated by unconsciously motivated accidents or injuries. While our discussion so far has focussed on the patients with the most pronounced pain vulnerability, we should keep in mind that there are also persons among whom the specific psychodynamic constellation conductive to pain may be activated on only a few occasions in their lives.

(1) *When external circumstances fail to satisfy the unconscious need to suffer:* We have already commented on the patient in whom pain develops when things begin to go well. These are always individuals with an exaggerated need to suffer who may remain relatively pain-free as long as external circumstances make life difficult. When the environment does not treat them harshly enough or they cannot get it to do so, it seems almost as if they inflict pain upon themselves.

A 45-year-old woman had at various times abdominal pain ("chronic appendicitis"), back pain, and finally severe pain in the left side of the jaw, left ear, and left side of the temple. She described the latter as "like a jab with an icepick." Although she came from a wealthy and socially prominent family, at the age of 25 she married a ne'er-do-well who cruelly mistreated her. She was humiliated by the divorce 3 years later. She remarried 12 years later and although this was a good marriage, it was marred by a series of distressing deaths, injuries, and illnesses in her family. In spite of the fact that small children irritated her, she adopted two little boys in rapid succession when she was over 40 years old. She was always getting sick. Her face pain began just at a time when things finally seemed to be going well for the first time, and after she had consented to allow her paralyzed mother-in-law, whose care she had undertaken at great personal sacrifice for many years, to go to a nursing home.

A 32-year-old woman, married to a brutal, alcoholic man who frequently beat her and the children, and who provided for her most inadequately, struggled hard to maintain herself. She began to suffer a series of painful disabilities when her husband underwent a religious conversion, gave up drinking, and became the model of a conscientious and considerate husband and father. Just when she had everything to live for, her pain prevented her from enjoying it.

Such precipitating circumstances are easily overlooked if the physician fails to recognize that for certain persons, success and good fortune are stressful in that they mobilize intolerable feelings of guilt (Freud, 1937/1950; Schuster, 1955). These persons really feel that they do not deserve happiness or success and they must suffer to achieve it.

(2) *As a response to a real, threatened, or fantasied loss:* Following the death or any permanent loss of a loved person, or during the period of anticipation of such a loss, the survivor may develop pain during the period of mourning and sometimes on anniversaries of the mourning. Szasz has pointed out how the mourner may take a part of his own body as a love object in place of the lost person and by experiencing pain in this part, symbolically assure himself of its continued presence (Szasz, 1957). He designates pain as an affect that warns of the danger or threat of loss of a body part. I agree with this formulation but find it incomplete, for it does not sufficiently include the affect of guilt. While following the loss of a loved person one becomes more self-centered and sometimes more aware of body sensations (or also at times less aware), this is not experienced as pain by the sufferer unless there is also a strong element of guilt, most often related to ambivalence toward the lost person. In a study of patients with ulcerative colitis we observed that if a relationship with a love object was threatened by some overt or unconscious aggressive act or fantasy and the patient re-

sponded with guilt, then pain (usually headache) developed; if the patient responded with feelings of despair, helplessness, or hopelessness, activation of the colitis was the more usual response (Engel, 1952).

A classic illustration of pain in response to a sudden loss is illustrated in the following case:

> A 42-year-old woman had a brief attack of sharp pain in the left anterior chest. In the interview she almost immediately began to speak of how upset she had been since the shotgun murder of her brother-in-law one week earlier. He was shot in the left side of the chest. His body was taken South for burial, but she had to remain home to care for the children. She cried when thinking or speaking of this event. She greatly admired and was very fond of this man who was a stable and successful man in the community. In contrast, her husband (the victim's brother) was irresponsible and abusive. In fact, exactly 1 year earlier, while drinking, he brutally beat her and then threatened to shoot her with a shotgun. She averted this by clutching her infant to her chest and jumping out the (ground-floor) window. She preferred charges against him and he was currently on probation. Further interviewing strongly indicated a guilty wish that the victim had been the husband rather than his brother.

While many episodes of pain occur in direct relationship to the loss of a loved person, as in this case, many more occur in relation to threatened losses, anniversaries of losses, or fantasied losses. Thus we may find pain developing in relationship to the illness or impending departure of important family members or friends, where the patient responds with, or had previously experienced aggressive feelings toward such persons. Or the patient may experience the loss or its anniversary as a painful reminder of guilt, and actually suffer with it in the form of pain.

(3) *When guilt is evoked by intense aggressive or forbidden sexual feelings:* There are some individuals for whom any expression of aggression is unacceptable and even the threat or possibility that aggression might be expressed provokes guilt. Some of these persons instead experience pain, sometimes without any aggression being expressed and sometimes remorsefully after it has been expressed. After the pain develops, the provoking situation may be forgotten or only vaguely remembered or the patient may recall it

remorsefully, consciously accepting the pain as a punishment and as a warning against future expressions of aggression. Some patients observe that their pains occur when they do not control themselves.

A 32-year-old woman, who also had had ulcerative colitis, was compulsively clean and always kept close rein on any expression of aggression. Her 2 1/2 year-old son defecated in his crib and smeared the feces. She became furious and immediately spanked him. A few hours later a severe headache developed. She felt remorseful for her outbreak of temper and resolved not to do so again. The headache was considered a deserved punishment.

When the provoking situation involves sexual impulses, these, in contrast to the aggressive impulses, are almost always at an unconscious level and must be inferred by the examiner. In general, they involve situations that might normally be expected to be sexually exciting, but are not so recognized by these patients, who instead experience pain; or more subtle situations in which the precipitating stimulus has special symbolic meaning to the individual, generally reminiscent of some childhood sexual conflict. Pains so experienced follow the classic model of the hysterical conversion mechanism, in which the pain simultaneously expresses symbolically the forbidden impulse and at the same time successfully prevents it being acted upon. When the conversion symptom is pain, we find that along with the sexual impulse there is always a strong aggressive component and guilt. The sexual fantasy is a sadomasochistic one.

A 26-year-old woman with a variety of hysterical manifestations had several episodes of pain and burning at the end of urination. The urine examination was always negative, but she referred to it as "my cystitis." One episode occurred during her first year of marriage. Her husband proved less capable sexually than she hoped for and she felt both frustrated and angry. As a child, the bathroom was the scene of many sexual fantasies and of masturbation, which included poking things in and around the urethra. The symptoms recurred briefly during the course of psychoanalysis when her husband had a severe case of flu and was sexually inattentive for several weeks. She developed fleeting sexual fantasies about the

analyst and then her "cystitis" recurred. The painful dysuria
promptly disappeared when these transference sexual feelings
were brought up during the analytic hour and connected with
the childhood fantasies and masturbatory activities.

The Location of the Pain

The patient usually describes the pain as occurring in some part of
his body, whether it originates there or not. When no peripheral
factor is operating, the patient still assigns a location to the pain.
This choice of site of the pain is determined by one or more of the
following:

(1) *A peripherally provoked pain experienced by the patient
sometime in the past:* In essence, the patient revives unconsciously
a past pain experience and by mechanisms not understood suffers
again from pain of the same character and in the same location as
the original pain. This may be the pain of a past injury, an operation, or any physical disorder that had occurred at a time when the
pain could fulfill, directly or indirectly, a psychic regulating role
for the patient. It may have been punishment or it may have been
the vehicle whereby a relationship was reestablished. Some postoperative and posttraumatic pain syndromes are of this sort.

A young man had repeated bouts of severe searing shocks
of pain in the right side of his forehead. These came on with
explosive suddenness, sometimes associated with a sensation
of flashing light and staggering, and were followed by a dull,
throbbing pain in growing intensity.

When he was 12 years old he prepared a home-made bomb, one
of numerous aggressive acts unconsciously directed toward his
stern and punitive father. The bomb exploded prematurely and he
suffered a depressed skull fracture as well as the loss of several fingers of his left hand. He felt extremely guilty and considered the
accident a deserved punishment. The location and character of the
head pain exactly duplicated the original accident. The pain characteristically occurred in settings in which anger toward authority
figures was blocked by guilt. Sometimes he could terminate the
pain by an attack of blind destructive fury against some inanimate
object, such as a piece of furniture.

The widest variety of painful disorders in the past may provide the
basis for future pain experiences and a careful history often will

uncover the original painful incident as well as the psychological factors operating at the time. When the current pain, which may be described in terms identical with the original pain, is not also accompanied by the appropriate physical or laboratory findings, especially when this occurs in a person with the other characteristics of the "pain-prone" population, the diagnosis is strongly suggested. This is illustrated by the patient with ear pain who in the past had otitis media; the patient with throat pain who once had a peritonsillar abscess; the patient with painful dysuria and frequency and normal urine who once had acute cystitis.

(2) *A pain actually experienced by someone else or a pain the patient imagined or wished the other person experienced:* This is perhaps the most common and the most important determinant of the site of the pain. It involves several important psychologic mechanisms. First of all, the other person is important to the patient and is one with whom the patient is in some (usually unconscious) conflict or from whom he has been or may be separated. Secondly, it involves the psychic mechanism of identification, meaning that the patient unconsciously becomes like the other person, notably in terms of suffering like him. We have already mentioned real, threatened, or fantasied losses and guilt for forbidden impulses as precipitating factors. We can now add that the location of pain may be determined by the real or fantasied location of pain in the other person(s). It must be emphasized that this is unconscious. The patient is unaware of the connection between his pain and the pain of the other person, and if directly questioned will never consciously make the connection, although he may unconsciously reveal it by word or gesture. On the other hand, if the physician meticulously explores the history of pain and illness of all the important persons in the patient's life, he will usually uncover without much difficulty the model for the patient's pain. To do this the patient is asked to describe the symptoms of each person, paying particular attention to the patient's idea of the pain.

A 42-year-old man complained of severe stabbing pain in the region of the left nipple. This occurred while he was out hunting and just taking aim at a buck deer. He felt fearful, had difficulty breathing, became lightheaded, and collapsed. The patient's father had died of a "heart attack" during the previous fall. The medical student who took the history as-

sumed that the patient know his father's pain had been sub-
sternal. When asked where his father's pain was, the patient
said, "I don't know," but he pointed to the region of his own
pain.

Sometimes we know the other person's illness to be painless, only
to discover the patient thought otherwise. Thus, edema of the an-
kles may be assumed to be painful, or dyspnea may be thought to
be an expression of pain. In such cases the patient may describe
the pain he believed the other person to have suffered in the same
terms he used to describe his own pain. There is little chance of
overlooking such relations if one always gets the patient's description. One may even ask, "What did you imagine it was like?" The
cases already noted have provided a number of examples of this
mechanism. The following cases offer additional data.

A 41-year-old unmarried woman, a teacher, lived with and
took care of her ailing mother for many years until her death 1
month before the beginning of the patient's face pain. She
slept in the same bed as her mother. On the night of her mother's death she had awakened to find that the right side of her
mother's face was drawn and a short time later it became blue.
She was breathing heavily and the patient *believed* her to be
suffering great pain. She called for help, but when unable to
secure any, climbed back into bed only to realize that her
mother was dead.

She had been engaged to a man for many years but had
not married because she could not leave her mother. However,
upon her mother's death, she first felt emancipated, and
bought a house, but then pain developed in the right side of
her face and because of it she gave up both her home and fi-
ance. She expressed remorse at her feelings of emancipation
after her mother's death and consciously considered the pain
as punishment, a sign that she was being inconsiderate of her
mother's memory.

A 47-year-old married woman had experienced strong
guilt when her only daughter was born 22 years ago with a
cleft palate and harelip. She felt that this was the result of her
husband's practice of coitus interruptus. When her doctor implied that this might have resulted from clumsy attempts at
abortion, she said, "That was just like a slap in the face to

me." The patient's mother also had indicated by innuendo that she believed her daughter was in some way responsible for the baby's defect. The mother suffered from erysipelas of the face 15 years ago and the patient took care of her. The mother has had face pain from time to time since then. The patient's face pain began 1 month after the daughter underwent the first of a long series of plastic operations on her face. The patient commented, "I am doing the suffering for her." The patient imagined that her daughter suffered great pain from these procedures, although actually this was not so.

In this last case we note how the choice of location may be overdetermined, here involving not only the daughter's facial deformity and operations, but also the "slap in the face" and the mother's erysipelas and face pain.

A 31-year-old married woman had severe pain in the right side of the neck and throat, radiating into the shoulder, right eye, and cheek. This had developed while she was taking care of her mother, who had suddenly acquired erysipelas of the face. It began while the patient was undergoing treatment from the chiropractor who was taking care of her mother and who had recommended a chiropractic treatment as a prophylactic measure. When asked what part of her mother's face was involved by the erysipelas, the patient was unable to recall, but placed her hand over the painful area of her own face.

Among other symptoms, a 23-year-old married woman had severe throbbing pain in the temporal regions radiating into the eyes. Her soldier husband had been injured in combat. He had sent her a photograph of himself in which he had cut out the left eye with scissors, indicating that this was the extent of his injury. The patient's symptoms began a week later. It developed that just before he went overseas she had learned that he had been involved in an extramarital affair. She was so angry that she struck him violently in the eye, knocking him down. Under pentothal hypnosis she told how much she wanted him punished. "I wanted him to get as much hurt as I was. I hoped he would get his leg or his foot, or his privates shot off." While he was overseas she had a brief affair, over which she felt very guilty. It was shortly after her lover had left her that she received the news of her husband's injury and the photograph. She was tremendously concerned at his possible retaliation for her infidelity and her pain began when she received word that he was being shipped home.

Sometimes the site of the pain is determined by a conscious or unconscious wish that the other person suffer pain. This may have appeared only as a fleeting thought or may not have been associated with the person at all. This is illustrative of the intrapsychic operation of lex talionis, the patient inflicting on himself exactly what he wished on the other person.

We can understand these determinants of pain location in terms of the importance of object relations (interpersonal relations) in the maintenance of health and of psychic balance. They are expressions *par excellence* of attempts to maintain object relations, albeit at a price. It is as if the patient says, "If I can't continue to have this relationship and get from it what I want and need, I will become like him in some way." This is a generally used mechanism to deal with a real or threatened loss, but in these cases, mainly because of guilt and the role of pain in past relationships, the patient experiences the object's pain, real or fantasied. By such a psychic experience of pain the patient simultaneously denies the intensity of the loss and atones for his guilt.

Psychiatric Diagnosis

While similar psychodynamic features may operate, these patients do not constitute a homogeneous group in terms of psychiatric nosology.

(1) *Conversion hysteria:* The largest number of these patients satisfy the requirements for the diagnosis of conversion hysteria, and their histories usually reveal many other conversion symptoms, such as globus, fainting, aphonia, sensory, or motor disturbances. They manifest the relative indifference to or exaggerated display of symptoms, as well as the dramatic, exhibitionistic, seductive, or shy behavior so common among hysteric persons. They are suggestible and may have intense emotional involvements with the physician, often associated with dramatic remissions and relapses of symptoms. To varying degrees they may have been involved in acting out behavior, including drinking, use of drugs, and sexual promiscuity. The men patients are often relatively passive and

have feminine identification, usually with the mother. A peculiarly intense interest and preoccupation with hunting, especially solitary hunting has, in my experience, been a common finding among the men. The hysterical patients with pain generally differ from those without pain in the prominence of sadistic and masochistic elements in their sexual developments, usually with pronounced guilt.

The following case is a classic example of conversion hysteria with pain as a prominent manifestation. It is presented in detail because patients with conversion hysteria constitute the largest percentage of the pain-prone population, and a thorough study of this case protocol will be richly rewarding in illustrating the characteristic features of hysterical patients with pain. Interpretative comments, in brackets, call attention to some of the characteristic features of psychogenic pain and the pain-prone patient discussed in the body of this paper.

A 27-year-old married woman, a singer by profession, had suffered from pain in her face and head for many years. She was first seen in February 1945. She felt she could distinguish at least three kinds of pain. At about the age of 11 or 12 she began to have attacks of pain in the right side of the face. This pain became extremely severe during a pregnancy that ended in a spontaneous abortion at 3 months in October 1944. The attacks usually began as a dull ache over the right eye, and rapidly progressed to a severe throbbing pain involving the entire side of the head and face and radiating into the neck and shoulder. This was associated with tearing of the right eye, stiffness of the right nostril, and at times flushing and hyperesthesia of the right side of the face. The pain was made worse by movement and noise, and when severe was associated with nausea and vomiting. Such attacks lasted a day or more.

A second type of face pain consisted of sudden brief shooting pain of moderate intensity involving the right cheek and followed by a dull aching pain. This pain had been present intermittently for about a year.

The third pain was of several years' duration and consisted of a sudden sharp, burning pain arising at the angle of the right jaw, radiating into the teeth, along the ramus, and into the ear. This pain generally came on when she was about to eat. It was associated with increased salivation. Generally it lasted several minutes and then subsided, permitting the patient to go on with her meal. She was examined for salivary duct calculus but none was found. Detailed examination, including neurologic, roentgen, and dental study, revealed no abnormalities.

At first the patient stated that her general health was and always had been good and that if it were not for the face pain she would be entirely well. It soon became evident that this was not so. She also suffered from attacks of nausea and vomiting; she was "sensitive" to many food items that induced nausea, vomiting and urticaria a few minutes after ingestion and sometimes simply on sight; she had attacks of bloating and swelling of the abdomen; she had shaking chills, with chattering of the teeth; and a subjective feeling of great coldness, during which her hands and feet would blanch and become icy cold; she had attacks of breathlessness, dizziness, and numbness and tingling, during which she occasionally lost consciousness; paroxysms of cough occurred that could not be explained on the basis of any respiratory tract disease, although she had had two to three attacks of rather typical bronchial asthma in her life; she had dyspareunia and was totally frigid; she suffered with urinary frequency and urgency. [Other hysterical conversion symptoms.]

The patient, an only child, was born in Chicago in 1918. Both parents were exceedingly neurotic persons. The mother was a successful business woman at the time of her marriage, although it was rumored that her success was partially accounted for by being the mistress of the employer. Unable to get him to marry her, she impulsively married her present husband as a spiteful gesture. He at this time was a rather inconsequential but handsome man, who so far had been quite unsuccessful in establishing himself as a business man. His wife paid his debts, set him up in business, and thereafter never permitted him to forget her role. For a period he was quite successful, but in 1928 he lost all his money and went heavily in debt. Since then he has held only small jobs and tends to use alcohol to a considerable degree. [Aggressive, controlling mother; relatively passive father.]

The patient felt the parents' marriage to be entirely devoid of any love or affection. They quarrelled frequently and violently. The patient always felt in the middle. She recalled one occasion when her mother threw a hammer at her father, and another occasion when he hit her mother with an ash tray. Not infrequently she had witnessed them strike each other in the face during quarrels. [Prominence of aggression in early family relations.] During such scenes the little girl felt she had to separate the two combatants "lest the quarrel end in murder." She consciously directed the parents' anger toward herself in order to avoid their hurting each other. On one occasion she scratched her father's face to "bring him to his senses." [As child, deflects aggression to herself.]

The patient said the mother avoided any sexual contact with father and, besides, she believed he was impotent anyway. "Mother could scare anyone into impotency." She was not born until the parents had been married 9 years, when they were 35 years old. The mother carried on a constant harangue against her father. She repeatedly warned the patient to have nothing to do with men, especially to avoid sexual contact. Even after the patient's marriage, her mother continued to urge her to have a separate bedroom as she herself had. [Mother's hostility to men and fear of sex.]

In 1938 the father was discovered to have cancer of the urinary bladder. The mother openly taunted him with the diagnosis and expressed pleasure that she would now be free of him. [Mother's sadism.] A subtotal cystectomy was performed and the father recovered, although he was left with frequency of urination. More recently the father had had a heart condition and was short of breath. [Factors in patient's "choice" of respiratory and urinary symptoms.]

During the early contacts with the patient she was most bitter toward her mother, whom she described as argumentative, domineering, nasty, and hypercritical, with no love for her. After such attacks on the mother, however, the patient would have the impulse to call her on the phone, and then would feel remorseful because her mother seemed more kind and interested than she had described her to be. [Hostility to mother, guilt, and submission.] On the other hand, she first described her father as "sweet and nice." He had beautiful curly hair and would let his little daughter play hairdresser and fuss with his hair for hours. Later on, statements changed and she said he was "wishy-washy, inconsistent, and an opportunist," that he "always disappointed me." "My dream castle is nothing but a backwoods shed," was her comment after a visit from father. [Disappointment with father.]

As a little girl she had tried to get close to her father, but her mother would never permit this. Mother would make fun of any show of affection between the two or would fly into a rage and accuse them of conspiring against her. On many occasions the mother threatened to leave home, and when father and daughter begged her to stay, she ridiculed them. Several times the mother spent all day in a movie to simulate such a threat. [Mother's sadism.] The little girl was heartbroken. Father always dealt with mother's threat by giving in. He wanted peace at any price.

The patient described herself as a difficult child to take care of. She devised various technics to provoke or exasperate her mother. One was to hide her mother's prized possessions, tell her she had hidden them, but not where. This generally led to a spanking. [Patient's use of pain and punishment as way of relating to mother.]

At a very early age she demonstrated unusual ability in singing. The mother had a "magnificent voice" and cultivated her little daughter's talent, functioning for a period as her teacher. When she was 9 she won a singing contest and made her debut with a nationally known symphony orchestra. Following the concert her mother pointed out that Mozart had made his debut at an earlier age. [Mother's depreciating and rivalrous attitudes.] Thereafter the patient concentrated on her singing, studied with well-known teachers, and made several public appearances. She progressed rapidly in school, finishing high school at 15, and college at 20. For a while in college she lost interest in a career as a singer; but after graduation she joined a light opera company that toured the country. She often had the leading soprano role and received good press notices. Her mother, however, always depreciated her performances.

Her early sexual education was very strict. Her mother depreciated all things sexual, and warned the child against any sexual activity. She kept her from wearing attractive or feminine clothing, opposed her fixing her hair, and insisted that she wear glasses although she had no need for them. In high school and college she was known as "Prudence Prim." Her mother would not permit her to go out alone until she was 21 years old, saying only bad girls went out. She was not permitted to live away from home. In early adolescence she fought hard to get away and mother let her go to boarding school. After a few months mother brought her home because she thought she was having too good a time. [Mother's depreciation of femininity and sexuality. The patient submits.] Her menses began at 11, 2 weeks after an auto accident (which will be described in detail later.) Although she had been told about menses, she thought they were the result of the accident.

The patient was married in August 1942. She has not previously gone out with many men, although she enjoyed their company on an intellectual basis. She liked to be with a group of men on a "man-to-man basis." She had had no sexual experience until marriage. [Patient's masculine identification and sexual inhibitions.] She had gone with her husband about 2 months when they became engaged; they were married 6 months later. He was in the army at that time and stationed near Boston awaiting embarkation. Immediately after the ceremony, coughing and wheezing developed that became so severe over the course of the next 2 weeks that she felt compelled to go home to Chicago. [Asthma in response to first real separation from mother.] As she stepped from the train and was met by her mother her asthma ceased and did not recur. The next day her husband was shipped overseas and she felt guilty that she was not there to see him off.

The patient worked in a war plant during her husband's absence and held a rather responsible position. She lived with her parents. In the Fall of 1943 her husband returned to the United States to convalesce from an attack of pleurisy and she joined him. In June 1944 she became pregnant and felt disgusted in spite of the fact that she had been trying to get pregnant for several months and was beginning to worry about sterility. During the pregnancy she had a great deal of nausea and vomiting and almost continuous severe head and face pain. She remained very active and "heaved furniture around." [Patient's self-destructive behavior.] Three months later she aborted while visiting her mother. She first felt very panicky and then became somewhat depressed. [Guilt.] She had the thought that she had not long to live and that her husband would be unhappy if she died. She behaved provocatively toward him and deliberately irritated him, ". . . so that he would hate me and would not miss me and could remarry." Several times she made the gesture of packing her bags and leaving. At other times she provoked the neighbors, sometimes by her singing, and she often got herself into unhappy situations with tradespeople and friends. [She provokes attacks on herself.]

During the period of therapy there occurred a number of experiences during sleep that her husband wrote down and brought in for discussion. The patient had complete amnesia for these experiences but was able to bring important associations. Two such episodes were particularly revealing:

(1) One night she said while asleep, "He hit me in the face with a buckle. I was a naughty girl." This recalled an incident at age 4. She had been naughty and mother insisted that father punish her. He was undressing. As he pulled his belt from his pants he suddenly struck her violently in the face with the buckle end. [Determinants of the face as location of pain.] "I remember hating him violently after that." Once, at 18, during a violent quarrel between the parents, the patient thought, "If he hits me, I would murder him." Just before her husband was discharged from the army she impulsively threw all his belts into an incinerator. They made her feel very uncomfortable, but as she watched them burn she had a happy feeling of triumph. This reminded her that mother had often used father's belt to strike her. [Unconscious association between father and husband. Aggression and guilt.]

Later she brought up that on two occasions she had provoked her husband to the extent that he had slapped her face. A severe exacerbation of face pain resulted on both occasions.

(2) The most dramatic episode concerned the auto accident to which she had briefly alluded in the first interview. At the time she merely said that she had been in an auto accident at age 11, and that she suffered a fractured kneecap and was in a cast for a year. She did not mention any injury suffered by mother. [First face pain began when the patient was 11 or 12.]

While asleep the patient tossed restlessly and began talking. [Reliving a traumatic episode.] "I know he didn't have any lights on. He turned them on after he got to the middle of the street. We never start to cross the street without looking." She cried out in pain, "My knee, my knee! That morphine makes me see the lights all over again. That car is rolling mother down the street and it isn't going to stop. I can't stand that car rolling her. I see her face full of blood. The eye is cut. She is dead. My face, my face, my face hurts." [Injury to mother's face as determinant of site of pain.] The patient beat on the bed. She awakened and appeared terrified. "I have to get up and see if I can walk." She struggled with her husband to get up, but was unable to. Her teeth chattered violently and she had a shaking chill at this point. "I am cold like I was sitting in the snow that night." The husband observed: "She was breathing rapidly and her arms and legs were icy cold. There was decided swelling of the right cheek that was red and hot over the area of pain. I sensed this temperature change by contrasting the two sides of the face. She writhed, clutched, and gasped, so intense was the pain. A cold object pressed against the pain area produced a shocking feeling in the face. "Light hurt her eyes." In referring to the shortness of breath, the patient commented, "It feels as if someone is sitting on my chest." [Origin of other conversion symptoms.]

The patient was then able to describe the accident in more detail. It occurred in a suburban district at night where it was quite deserted. It was a cold wintry night, 13°F below zero, with snow on the ground. Mother and daughter stepped from the streetcar and started to cross the street. Suddenly they realized a car without lights was bearing down on them. Just before striking, the headlights were turned on and glared in their eyes. Mother raised her hand to protect her face. She was struck by the car and dragged half a block. The patient was knocked to her knees and found herself alone in the dark, sitting in the snow. She screamed; she felt alone and deserted. She shivered with the cold and it seemed endless before anyone picked her up. When she saw her mother, her face looked "like someone had beaten it with a hammer." Mother was coughing up blood. The patient was brought to a hospital where she received morphine and had repetitive frightening dreams of the accident. Her mother, who recovered quickly, brought violets, which remain the patient's favorite flower. The patient remained in a cast for a year and was taken care of at home by her mother. She described this as a not unhappy time. "I was completely helpless. Whenever I have been ill, mother has been good to me." [Love from mother when she suffered.]

(2) *Depression:* Another group of patients suffers predominantly from depression. The generally depressed appearance, the retarded or agitated behavior, the content of speech, the expressed affects of sadness, guilt and shame, all identify the depression and this is usually documented by history. Some patients, it will be found, have had previous episodes of depression without pain and some are the chronically gloomy and depressive characters already described. A common error by the physician is to assume that the patient is depressed because he has pain. Investigation will usually make clear that the experience of pain serves to attenuate the guilt and shame of the depression. Indeed, in some instances the pain is clearly protecting the patient from more intense depression and even suicide. This group of patients in particular may become addicted to drugs.

(3) *Hypochondriasis:* The hypochondriacal patient experiences and communicates his pain or other body sensations in a distinctive way. One quickly notes its peculiarly intense and persistent quality. It may not be as severe as it is inescapable, annoying, and bedeviling, and the patient is made desperate by the pain. As the physician listens to the patient's description he immediately notes the urgency with which the patient seeks relief and his tremendous concern as to what the pain means. He often seems more concerned with the interpretation of the pain—is it cancer or some terrible infection—then with the pain *per se*, and he is little or not at all reassured by the doctor's examinations. There is often a distinct quality of being persecuted by the pain. At the same time it will be found that the patient lavishes all varieties of attention and care on the painful part, somewhat in contrast to the relative indifference of the hysteric patient or the long-suffering attitude of the depressive patient. Some of these patients are prepsychotic.

(4) *Schizophrenia:* Closely related to the hypochondriacal patients are those who are psychotic and whose pain represents a delusion. Many of these patients are not recognized as psychotic simply because their complaint is pain. But the alert physician will note the following qualities. The patient truly feels persecuted by his pain and seeks help with a desperation that is impressive. It is not so much that it is painful as that it is unrelenting, annoying,

and inescapable. The description of the pain may include bizarre ideas that are expressed as vivid analogies or as actualities. A pregnant woman had pain in the lower part of her abdomen. She ascribed this to being poked by the erect penis of her unborn child who she knew was a boy. Little further inquiry was needed to establish the diagnosis of schizophrenia. Patients express convictions that certain extraordinary changes have taken place in their bodies, the very bizarreness of which makes their delusional quality evident. A 55-year-old man with repeated attacks of abdominal pain said with conviction that his intestines were "twisted like a mop" and had to be untwisted, and begged for surgery. He also was convinced that there was some strange object in his abdomen, perhaps left in during previous surgery. Such patients usually manifest other paranoid qualities, including suspicious accusations against other physicians as being responsible for the pain. Or they may ascribe the pain to various outside influences, including rays and vibrations. A very important clinical point is the patient's tendency to associate the pain with nasal or rectal difficulties. Indeed these patients often first approach otolaryngologists or proctologists, or they may have sought treatment with colonic or nasal irrigations. The diagnosis will rarely be overlooked if the patient is given sufficient opportunity to present his explanation for the pain. This usually proves to be a complicated delusional concept.

It is perhaps important to mention here that often the schizophrenic patient experiences no pain or does not complain of it when an ordinary painful disorder develops. An acute coronary occlusion or a perforated appendix may be entirely silent as far as the observer is concerned. Actually, pain is experienced in a delusional fashion by the schizophrenic relatively infrequently.

Summary

The general principles formulated in this paper may be summarized as follows:

1. What is experienced and reported as pain is a psychological phenomenon. Pain does not come into being without the operation of the psychic mechanisms that give rise to its iden-

tifiable qualities and that permit its perception. In neuro-physiological terms this also means there is no pain without the participation of higher nervous centers.

2. Developmentally, however, pain evolves from patterns of impulses arising from peripheral receptors that are part of the basic biologic nociceptive system for the protection of the organism from injury. The psychic experience, pain, develops phylogenetically and ontogenetically from what was originally only a reflex organization. This may be compared to the necessity for functioning eyes and ears to receive light and sound waves before the complex psychic experiences of seeing and hearing can evolve.

3. Once the psychic organization necessary for pain has evolved, the experience, pain, no longer requires peripheral stimulation to be provoked, just as visual and auditory sensations (hallucinations) may occur without sense organ input. When such are projected outside the mind (in contrast to a painful thought or a painful frame of mind) they are felt as being in some part of the body and are to the patient indistinguishable from pain arising in the periphery.

4. Since the experience, pain, and the sensory experiences from which it evolves are part of the biologic equipment whereby the individual learns about the environment and about his body, and since this has a special function as a warning or indicator of damage to body parts, pain plays an important role in the total psychologic development of the individual. Indeed, pain, along with other affects, comes to occupy a key position in the regulation of the total psychic economy. We discover that in the course of the child's development, pain and relief of pain enter into the formation of interpersonal (object) relations and into the concepts of good and bad, reward and punishment, success and failure. Pain becomes par excellence a means of assuaging guilt and thereby influences object relationships.

5. From the clinical viewpoint we discover that disordered neural patterns originating in the periphery confer certain qualities on the pain experience that permit the physician to recognize their presence and hence make a presumptive diagnosis of an organic lesion.

6. Clinical psychological studies of all varieties of patients

with pain reveal that some individuals are more prone than others to use pain as a psychic regulator, whether the pain includes a peripheral source of stimulation or not. These pain-prone individuals usually show some or all of the following features:

- A prominence of conscious and unconscious guilt, with pain serving as a relatively satisfactory means of atonement.
- A background that tends to predispose to the use of pain for such purposes.
- A history of suffering and defeat and intolerance of success (masochistic character structure). A propensity to solicit pain, as evidenced by the large number of painful injuries, operations and treatments.
- A strong aggressive drive that is not fulfilled, pain being experienced instead.
- Development of pain as a replacement for a loss at times when a relationship is threatened or lost.
- A tendency toward a sadomasochistic type of sexual development, with some episodes of pain occurring in settings of conflict over sexual impulses.
- A location of pain determined by unconscious identification with a love object, the pain being one suffered by the patient himself when in some conflict with the object, or a pain suffered by the object in fact or in the patient's fantasy.
- Psychiatric diagnoses include conversion hysteria, depression, hypochondriasis, and paranoid schizophrenia, or mixtures of these. Some patients with pain do not fit into any distinct nosologic category.

Conclusion

I would like to close with a historical note. It is astonishing how little discussions of pain in standard textbooks of medicine have changed in a hundred years. In a textbook published in 1858, Wood discusses pain in terms which differ only in details from what appears in Harrison's *Principles of Internal Medicine*, published in 1954 (Wood, 1858; Harrison, 1954). These details mainly concern more recent knowledge about the anatomy and physiology of nerve pathways. In both sources it is taken for granted that pain arises from the periphery or in the nerves themselves. The most modern explanation of chronic pain is that recurring painful stimuli from the periphery set up reverberating circuits related to the central activating system which influence, and are in turn influenced by, the cerebral cortex so that there may develop a syndrome or chronic pain (Von Magen, 1957)." In all these writings, psychological processes are relegated to a purely subsidiary role, such as reinforcing the reverberating circuit, or are simply dismissed by saying that the neurotic (or, in 1858, the "nervous") patient is less tolerant of or has a lower threshold for pain—clearly a cultural prejudice for which there is no scientific evidence. It is all the more remarkable that this state of affairs should continue to exist when, as early as 1895, Breuer and Freud in *Studies on Hysteria* published detailed case histories demonstrating convincingly pain as a psychogenic manifestation (1895/1955). In contrast to much of Freud's later writings, this early work includes a wealth of case material. The modern physician, regardless of his knowledge of or attitudes toward psychoanalysis, will find it richly rewarding to read these case histories, for in them he can learn for himself the nature of the data and observations that permitted Freud to discover how pain may develop as a purely psychic phenomenon. Freud himself was not primarily interested in pain, but it happened that among many of these patients pain was a common and prominent manifestation, as were a great number of other somatic symptoms that also proved to represent hysterical conversions. Indeed, one might be justified in saying that psychoanalysis came into being through the clarification of mechanism of some of these mysterious pain syndromes.

This leads to an interesting question: namely, how is it that this contribution to the understanding of pain has had so little influence on medicine in general, even on psychoanalysis. I believe the explanation is to be found in the peculiarities of medical practice. Freud began his practice as a neurologist and, in Vienna in the 1880's, undiagnosed pains were considered to be forms of neuralgia, an affection of nerves, concerning which the neurologist was the expert. As long as Freud was known primarily as a neurologist and his technic was not recognized as a form of psychotherapy, many such patients were referred to him and most went willingly enough. As he evolved into a psychoanalyst and the technic of treatment became increasingly recognized as a psychological one, there must have occurred a change in the categories of patients who were considered suitable for referral. Further, patients with conversion hysteria, who suffer primarily from somatic symptoms, are reluctant to seek psychological help. In general, they regard their symptoms as organic in origin, a belief in which they are often supported by their physicians. The pain patients in particular are among the most reluctant to accept a psychiatric referral, and to participate in psychotherapy if they do so. As time went on, Freud's practice consisted more and more on patients with the classic neurosis and with few exceptions this trend away from patients with somatic symptoms, including conversion hysteria, has continued to date. It is of interest in this respect that in Freud's early works, pain is referred to frequently, but later on one rarely finds any mention of pain. In the current scene, the analyst or psychiatrist is rarely consulted directly by a patient because of pain and only infrequently are such patients referred, and when they are many do not accept the referral. Thus the analyst and psychiatrist have had little opportunity to study this problem, which remains as common and difficult as ever. A large percentage of patients who consult physicians of all types belong to the group of "pain-prone" patients and are seeking help for painful disorders such as I have described in this paper.

This brings me also to the technic of investigation of these patients. Again, let me refer back to the original case histories of Breuer and Freud. These patients were not psychoanalyzed in the sense that we now understand the term. Every physician is free to rediscover for himself what Freud discovered about pain if he follows two simple principles: permit the patients to talk freely and take seriously what the patient says. If, in addition, he has some understanding of the psychic function of pain as I have outlined it in this paper, he will have no difficulty in confirming the observations of Freud as well as of those who followed him. This is not the place to discuss *in extenso* the technic of medical interview. Suffice it to say that an interview technic that permits the patient to speak of himself, his family, and his relationships as well as of his symptoms, which does not force a separation between what is regarded as organic and what is regarded as psychological or social, will be tremendously productive in clarifying the patient's illness. We have learned now that when one knows what one is looking for, this can be accomplished in a remarkably brief time. I have seen some patients in whom the basic dynamics of the pain, including an explanation of the choice of the pain and its location, could be worked out in as little time as 30 minutes; with a great number of patients an hour's interview will suffice. But even when more interview time than this is required, this is more economical in time and expense for both the physician and the patient than the currently traditional technic of "ruling out organic disease" and attempting to establish a diagnosis by exclusion. Such interminable diagnostic procedures may not only be a waste of time and money, but may also render virtually impossible the establishment of correct diagnosis simply because the patient himself becomes increasingly oriented towards this type of approach and less spontaneous in revealing personal and psychological data that the physician, by his approach and behavior, has made him feel are completely out of place. Needless to say, the physician whose technic of interview does not permit the patient spontaneously to reveal personal and psychological data along with his symptoms will not succeed in confirming the observations reported in this paper. But, for that matter, will the physician who uses only sabouraud's medium to examine urethral discharges succeed in confirming the relationship between the gonococcus and some case of gonorrhea. As in all matters scientific, the application of the appropriate method is indispensable.

References

Beecher, H. K. (1956). Limiting factors in experimental pain. *Journal of Chronic Diseases, 4*, 11.

Breuer, J. & Freud, S. (1895/1955). Studies on Hysteria. *Standard edition complete psychological works of Sigmund Freud*, London: Hogarth.

Eisele, C. W., Slee, V. N., & Hoffman, R. G. (1956). Can the practice of internal medicine be evaluated? *Ann. Internal Medicine, 44*, 144.

Engel, G. L. (1951). Primary atypical facial neuralgia: An hysterical conversion symptom. *Psychosomatic Medicine, 12*, 375.

Engel, G. L. (1956). Studies of ulcerative colitis. *iv*. The significance of headaches. *Psychosomatic Medicine, 18*, 334.

Freud, S. (1937/1950). Analysis. Terminable and Interminable. *Collected Works, vol. 5*. London: Hogarth.

Gooddy, Wu. (1957). On the nature of pain. *Brain 80*, 118.

Harrison, T. R. (1954). *Principles of internal medicine, 2nd ed.* New York: Blakiston.

Hart, H. (1957). Displacement guilt and pain. *Psychoanalytic Review, 34*, 259.

Kolb, L. C. (1954) *The painful phantom: psychology, physiology, and treatment.* American Lecture Series. Springfield, Il., Charles C. Thomas.

Libman, E. (1934). Observations on individual sensitiveness to pain with special reference to abdominal disorders. *Journal of American Medical Association, 102,* 335.

Osmond, H. (1957). A review of the clinical effects of psychotomimetic agents. *Ann. New York Academy Science, 66,* 418.

Penfield, W. & Jasper, H. (1954). *Epilepsy and the functional anatomy of the human brain.* Boston: Little, Brown.

Rangell, L. (1953). Psychiatric aspects of pain. *Psychosomatic Medicine, 15,* 22.

Rosen H. (1951). The hypnotic and hyponotherapeutic control of severe pain. *American Journal of Psychiatry 107,* 917.

Schilder, P. (1935). *The image and appearance of the human body.* London: Kegan, Paul, Trench, Trubner.

Schuster, D. (1955). On the fear of success. *Psychiatric Quart., 29,* 412–420.

Solomon, P., Leiderman, P. H., Mendelson, J. & Wexler, D. (1957). Sensory deprivation. A review. *American Journal of Psychiatry, 114,* 357.

Szasz, T. (1957). *Pain and pleasure.* New York: Basic Books.

Von Hagen, K. O. (1957). Chronic intolerable pain. *Journal of American Medical Association, 165,* 773.

Wolff, H. G. (1948). *Headache and other head pain.* New York. Oxford Univ. Press.

Wood, G. B. A. (1858). *A treatise on the practice of Medicine.* Philadelphia: Lippincott.

Index

Springer Publishing Company

PSYCHOLOGY AND HEALTH
Second Edition

Donald A. Bakal, PhD

Revised edition of *Psychology and Medicine*. This easily accessible work updates the author's approach to behavioral medicine, with examinations of mind–body integration, emotions, stress, psychopharmacology, pain—and much more.

Praise for the First Edition

"This accomplished book gives a convincing account of the inextricable interaction between mind and body in health and illness.... It is a study of immense width and depth...not averse to challenging accepted theories. This book is certainly the ultimate in the patient-centered, holistic approach." —**Nursing Times**

"...this approach has something to contribute to practically all aspects of medical practice...may be read with profit by all practitioners and students of the various caring professions." —**British Medical Journal**

Partial Contents:

Integrating Body and Mind • Psychobiology and Holistic Experience • Traditional Psychosomatic Theory • Signs, Symptoms, and Somatization

Emotions • Peripheral Determinants of Feeling • Brain Processes • Bio-Psycho-Social Approaches • Clinical Anxiety and Panic

Understanding Stress • Transactional Model • Bodily Responses and Individuality • Social Support: Cause or Consequence? • Sleep Disturbance: Insomnia • Psychological Stress and Surgery • Stress Management Training

Psychopharmacology: Mood Disorders and Addictions • Drugs and Psychobiology • Modes of Drug Action • Tricylic Medications • Placebo and Double-Blind Design • Somatic-Cognitive Interface in Depression • Relapse Prevention Model

Pain • Complexity of Pain • Physiological Mechanisms • Psychology of Pain Tolerance • Childbirth Labor Pain • Migraine and Daily Tension Headache • Cancer Pain

1992   256pp   0-8261-7900-2   hardcover

536 Broadway, New York, NY 10012-3955 • (212) 431-4370 • Fax (212) 941-7842

Springer Publishing Company

PERSONALITY AND ADVERSITY

Psychospiritual Aspects of Rehabilitation

Carolyn L. Vash, PhD

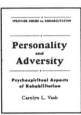

The author draws on her own experiences as a person with severe disabilities to bring us her newest textbook, Personality and Adversity. The main theme of this new work centers on adversity as a catalyst for psychospiritual growth. Using her artistic creativity, the author incorporates ideas from philosophy, religion, literature, and art to provide effective strategies for coping with disabilities.

Contents:

I: Observations and Findings. Adversity Strikes • Coping With Adverse Consequences • A Psychospiritual Dimension

II: Theoretical Constructs and Measures. Human Nature and Woundedness • Uses of Adversity • Templates of the Self

III: Implications and Suggestions. Discovery, Verification, and Education • Helping Ourselves and Each Other • Personality and Catastrophe: Partners in the Dance

Springer Series on Rehabilitation

1994   304pp   0-8261-8040-X   hardcover

536 Broadway, New York, NY 10012-3955 • (212) 431-4370 • Fax (212) 941-7842